Dr. Sebi

Encyclopedia of Herbs

The Complete Collection of Healing Herbs to Easily
Cleanse & Rejuvenate Your

Body and Achieve a Radiant

Lifelong Well Being

SIMON JR. JACKSON

Table of Contents

Introduction

Dr. Sebi, whose real name was Alfredo Bowman, was a self-proclaimed healer and herbalist who gained a following in the United States and beyond with his claims that he could cure a variety of diseases using a specific diet and herbal remedies. He was born in Honduras in 1933 and later moved to the United States.

Dr. Sebi believed that disease was caused by an excess of mucus in the body, and that his diet, which he called the "African Bio Mineral Balance," could eliminate mucus and restore health. The diet was based on the consumption of alkaline, plant-based foods and the avoidance of acidic foods, dairy, and meat.

He claimed that his diet could cure a variety of diseases, including cancer, diabetes, and AIDS. However, there is little scientific evidence to support these claims, and many of his recommendations have been criticized by medical professionals and nutrition experts.

The Dr. Sebi's diet is a big advocate of using natural remedies and herbs. Dr. Sebi's diet emphasizes the consumption of natural, plant-based foods and the use of herbal remedies as a way to support the body's natural healing mechanisms. This approach is based on the belief that the body is capable of healing itself if given the right conditions and nutrients.

He believed that synthetic drugs and other chemical interventions can disrupt the body's natural healing mechanisms and cause more harm than good. Instead, he advocated for the use of natural remedies, such as herbs and plant-based supplements, which he believed could help to support the body's natural healing processes without causing harmful side effects.

Dr. Sebi believed that many of the chronic diseases that afflict modern society are caused by poor diet and lifestyle choices, and that these conditions can be reversed through changes in diet and the use of natural remedies.

Keeping that in mind, this book is a comprehensive guidebook that explores the benefits of using natural remedies to support health and wellness. In this book, the I discus the advantages of natural remedies over synthetic medicines and explain how they can help to promote healing and prevent disease.

The book also delves into the Dr. Sebi diet and its focus on alkaline, plant-based foods and herbal remedies. It provides a detailed overview of the essential herbs used in the Dr. Sebi diet and explains how they can support the body's natural healing mechanisms.

With clear and concise explanations, this book is an essential resource for anyone looking to support their health and wellness with natural remedies. Whether you are new to natural remedies or an experienced practitioner, this book is sure to help you in the long run!

Chapter 1:
Introduction To Alkaline Healing Herbs

Exploring The History Of Alkaline Herbs

The use of herbs for medicinal purposes dates back to ancient civilizations, with evidence of herbal remedies found in Egyptian, Greek, Chinese, and Indian cultures. Using herbs for their alkaline properties to heal the body is a recent development. It can be traced back to the teachings of Dr. Sebi.

Dr. Sebi, whose real name was Alfredo Bowman, was a self-taught herbalist who developed an alkaline plant-based diet and a line of herbal supplements to treat various health conditions. He believed many diseases were caused by mucus buildup in the body and could be cured by consuming a diet of alkaline foods and herbs.

Dr. Sebi's philosophy and teachings gained popularity in the 1980s and 1990s, particularly in the African American and Hispanic communities. He claimed to have cured several chronic diseases using his alkaline diet and herbal remedies. His teachings and herbal products continue to be used today by those who follow an alkaline diet and lifestyle.

The evolution of alkaline herbs has continued beyond Dr. Sebi's teachings, with many herbalists and health practitioners advocating for using alkaline herbs to promote overall health and prevent disease. The popularity of alkaline herbs has also led to increased research and study of their potential health benefits, with new herbs being discovered and added to the list of alkaline healing herbs.

What Are Alkaline Herbs?

Alkaline healing herbs are plants with a high pH level and are known to help balance the body's acidity levels. These herbs are often used worldwide in traditional medicine to treat various ailments and promote overall wellness. The alkaline properties of these herbs make them beneficial for restoring the body's natural pH balance, which is essential for optimal health.

Some popular alkaline healing herbs include burdock root, sea moss, Irish moss, yellow dock, and sarsaparilla. These herbs are believed to have various health benefits, such as improving digestion, reducing inflammation, boosting immunity, and promoting detoxification. They can be consumed in various forms, such as teas, supplements, tinctures, and topical creams.

Using alkaline healing herbs has gained popularity recently as people seek natural and holistic approaches to health and wellness. These herbs offer a natural and effective way to support the body's natural healing processes without the side effects often associated with synthetic medications. Individuals can promote their health and well-being by incorporating alkaline healing herbs into their diets and lifestyles.

Understanding The Importance Of Alkaline Herbs

Alkaline herbs are essential in maintaining the body's pH balance and overall health. They are a rich source of essential vitamins, minerals, and other nutrients crucial for the proper functioning of the body's systems. By consuming alkaline herbs, we can help neutralize and reduce the harmful effects of excess acidity in our bodies, a common problem due to the highly acidic nature of modern diets.

Alkaline herbs can also help to improve our immune system by providing the body with antioxidants and anti-inflammatory compounds, which can help to reduce inflammation and promote healing. They can also help to reduce the risk of chronic diseases such as heart disease, cancer, and diabetes by providing the body with essential nutrients that support healthy organ function.

Furthermore, alkaline herbs can help to improve digestion and elimination, which are crucial for maintaining a healthy gut microbiome. They can also help to improve the absorption and utilization of essential nutrients, which can enhance overall health and well-being. Additionally, many alkaline herbs have natural detoxifying properties that can help to remove harmful toxins and other harmful substances from the body, promoting overall wellness and longevity.

The Different Usage Of Alkaline Herbs

In modern times, alkaline herbs have gained much attention due to their potential health benefits. Many now turn to natural remedies and traditional medicine to support their well-being. Alkaline herbs have become increasingly popular for their therapeutic properties. These herbs have been used for centuries in traditional medicine. They are now being studied for their potential to prevent and treat various health conditions.

One of the main reasons for the popularity of alkaline herbs is their potential to promote a healthy pH balance in the body. The human body is naturally slightly alkaline, with a pH of around 7.4. However, many modern diets and lifestyles can lead to an acidic environment in the body, which can be detrimental to health. Alkaline herbs are believed to help restore the body's natural pH balance, which can have a range of health benefits, including improved digestion, increased energy, and reduced inflammation.

Alkaline herbs are also rich in vitamins, minerals, and antioxidants, essential for overall health and well-being. Many of these herbs have been shown to have anti-inflammatory, antibacterial, and antiviral properties, which can help protect the body against infections and diseases. Additionally, some alkaline herbs are known to support specific systems in the body, such as the immune system, cardiovascular System, and nervous System.

Chapter 2:
Using Alkaline Herbs For Medical Conditions And More

What Is Alkalinity And What Happens If Your Body Becomes Acidic?

Alkalinity is a term used to describe being alkaline or having a high pH level. The pH scale ranges from 0 to 14, with 7 being neutral, anything below 7 being acidic, and anything above 7 being alkaline. Maintaining an alkaline internal condition is essential for good health and well-being.

What is the pH Value?

The pH value is a measure of the acidity or alkalinity of a substance. The pH scale ranges from 0 to 14, with 7 being neutral, anything below 7 being acidic, and anything above 7 being alkaline. The pH value of different parts of the body can vary. For example, the stomach has a pH value of around 2, which is highly acidic. In contrast, the blood has a pH value of around 7.4, which is slightly alkaline.

How pH Affects our Internal system

The pH of the body is important for maintaining normal bodily functions. The body has several mechanisms to regulate the pH levels, such as the kidneys and lungs. When the body's pH level becomes too acidic or too alkaline, it can lead to health problems. For example, when the pH level of the blood becomes too acidic, it can cause respiratory acidosis, a condition in which the body cannot remove enough carbon dioxide.

Why Maintain an Alkaline Internal Condition

Maintaining a balanced alkaline state within the body is crucial for optimal health and vitality. An overly acidic environment can give rise to multiple health issues such as inflammation, cancer, and bone degeneration. Incorporating alkaline-rich foods and plants can help stabilize the body's pH, minimizing the potential for these ailments. Furthermore, a more alkaline internal state can enhance energy, fortify the immune system, and elevate general well-being.

Benefits of an Alkaline Internal Condition

Having an internal alkaline balance can offer numerous health advantages, such as enhanced digestion, heightened energy, and diminished inflammation. Foods and herbs with alkaline properties are packed with essential vitamins, minerals, and antioxidants that can boost general health and vitality. Furthermore, these alkaline-rich foods and plants can bolster the performance of the liver and kidneys, the primary organs responsible for detoxifying the body.

The Different Health Conditions

Alkaline herbs have been recognized for their wide array of health benefits and have traditionally been employed for numerous medical ailments over the centuries. These plants are rich in antioxidants and possess potent anti-inflammatory capabilities, playing a vital role in preventing and addressing various health issues. Here are some ailments that can be alleviated with the use of alkaline herbs:

I. Acid Reflux: This condition arises when gastric acid reverses into the esophagus, leading to heartburn and discomfort. Herbs like ginger, turmeric, and fennel have properties that can mitigate the symptoms of acid reflux. For instance, ginger can enhance digestion and lower stomach lining inflammation, helping ward off acid reflux. Similarly, turmeric can ease esophagus inflammation, and fennel can curb stomach acid production and relieve heartburn.

II. Arthritis: This ailment induces inflammation within the joints, resulting in pain, rigidity, and swelling. Turmeric and ginger are alkaline herbs known to relieve arthritis symptoms due to their anti-inflammatory benefits. Specifically, turmeric houses a substance named curcumin, recognized for its capacity to diminish inflammation and joint discomfort. Ginger can further ease inflammation and promote joint flexibility.

III. High Blood Pressure: This is characterized by the excessive force of blood pressing against arterial walls. Alkaline plants like garlic and hawthorn can be beneficial in managing elevated blood pressure levels. Garlic is rich in a substance called allicin, which has proven efficacy in blood pressure reduction. Concurrently, hawthorn can expand blood vessels and optimize blood circulation, thereby assisting in regulating blood pressure.

IV. Insomnia: Individuals with insomnia struggle to fall or remain asleep. Alkaline herbs, including valerian root and passionflower, can enhance sleep patterns and curb insomnia. Valerian root is recognized for its calming effects that can facilitate sleep, while passionflower has demonstrated its potential to elevate sleep quality and diminish insomnia instances.

V. Respiratory Infections: These are ailments that compromise the respiratory apparatus, such as the flu, common cold, and bronchitis. Thyme and oregano are alkaline herbs that can be employed in addressing respiratory infections. Thyme has thymol, a compound with antiseptic and antibacterial qualities suited for respiratory infection treatment. Likewise, oregano boasts both antiviral and antibacterial traits that make it effective against respiratory infections.

VI. Digestive Complications: Problems like constipation, bloating, and diarrhea can be managed with alkaline herbs, including chamomile and peppermint. Peppermint can foster improved digestion and diminish bloating, whereas chamomile can lower digestive tract inflammation and bolster digestion.

VII. Depression and Anxiety Depression and anxiety are conditions that affect millions of people around the world. Alkaline herbs such as lavender and lemon balm can help to reduce symptoms of depression and anxiety. Lavender is an herb that has calming and relaxing properties and can help to reduce anxiety and improve mood. Lemon balm is another herb that can help to reduce anxiety and improve cognitive function.

VIII. Skin Conditions Skin conditions such as acne, eczema, and psoriasis can be treated with alkaline herbs such as aloe vera and calendula. Aloe vera is an anti-inflammatory and antiseptic herb that can help treat acne and other skin conditions. Calendula is another herb that has anti-inflammatory properties and can help to soothe and heal the skin.

IX. Headaches and Migraines Headaches and migraines can be treated with alkaline herbs such as feverfew and peppermint. Feverfew is an herb shown to reduce the frequency and severity of migraines. Peppermint is another herb that can help reduce tension headaches and migraines by improving blood flow and inflammation.

X. Allergies Allergies are a condition that occurs when the immune system overreacts to certain substances, causing symptoms such as runny nose, watery eyes, and itching. Alkaline herbs such as nettle and ginger can help to reduce allergy symptoms. Nettle is an herb that has antihistamine properties and can help to reduce allergy symptoms. Ginger is another herb that can help to reduce inflammation in the nasal passages and improve breathing.

XI. Diabetes Diabetes is a condition that occurs when the body is unable to regulate blood sugar levels. Alkaline herbs such as cinnamon and fenugreek can help to regulate blood sugar levels and improve insulin sensitivity. Cinnamon is an herb shown to improve blood sugar levels by increasing insulin sensitivity. Fenugreek is another herb that can help to regulate blood sugar levels and improve glucose tolerance.

Using Alkaline Herbs For Culinary

Alkaline herbs are considered to have an alkalizing effect on the body. These herbs are rich in minerals and nutrients that can help balance the body's pH levels, essential for good health and well-being. In addition to their health benefits, alkaline herbs are commonly used in cooking due to their unique flavors and culinary properties. In this section, we will explore the different culinary uses of alkaline herbs.

Flavor Enhancers

One of the main uses of alkaline herbs in cooking is as a flavor enhancer. Alkaline herbs such as basil, thyme, and oregano are commonly used to flavor various dishes, including soups, stews, and sauces. These herbs can be used fresh or dried and add a subtle or bold flavor to dishes depending on the amount used. The unique flavors of these herbs can also complement the flavors of other ingredients in a dish, making them a versatile addition to any recipe.

Natural Preservatives

Another use of alkaline herbs in cooking is as a natural preservative. Alkaline herbs such as rosemary and sage are known for their antioxidant and antibacterial properties, which can help to prevent food spoilage and extend the shelf life of foods. These herbs can be added to marinades, rubs, and other seasoning blends to help preserve the flavor and quality of the food.

Health Boosters

In addition to their culinary uses, alkaline herbs are known for their health benefits. Alkaline herbs such as ginger and turmeric are commonly used to boost the immune system and reduce inflammation. These herbs can be used in various dishes, including smoothies, soups, and stir-fries. The unique flavors of these herbs can add a spicy and warming flavor to dishes while also providing health benefits.

Color Enhancers

Alkaline herbs such as parsley and cilantro are commonly used as color enhancers in dishes. These herbs can add a bright green color to dishes, making them visually appealing and appetizing. They can be used as a garnish or added to sauces and dips to enhance the color and flavor of the dish.

Aromatics

Alkaline herbs are also commonly used as aromatics in cooking. Aromatics such as garlic, onion, and leeks are commonly used to add flavor and aroma to dishes. These herbs can be sautéed or roasted and add a rich and savory flavor to various dishes.

Culinary Herbs

Finally, alkaline herbs are commonly used as culinary herbs in cooking. Culinary herbs such as basil, thyme, and sage are commonly used to flavor various dishes. These herbs can be used fresh or dried and add a subtle or bold flavor to dishes depending on the amount used. They are often used in Italian and Mediterranean cuisine. They can be used in various dishes, including soups, stews, and sauces.

Using Alkaline Herbs Of Beauty And Skincare

Alkaline herbs are useful in cooking and maintaining internal health; they also have a range of beauty and skincare benefits. Many alkaline herbs contain essential oils, antioxidants, and other beneficial compounds that can help to nourish the skin and promote a healthy complexion. In this section, we will explore alkaline herbs' different beauty and skincare uses.

Skin Cleansers

One of the main uses of alkaline herbs in skin care is as a skin cleanser. Alkaline herbs such as rosemary and thyme are known for their antibacterial and antifungal properties, which can help to purify the skin and prevent acne breakouts. These herbs can be used to make a skin toner or added to facial steam to help cleanse and detoxify the skin.

Exfoliants

Another use of alkaline herbs in skincare is as an exfoliant. Alkaline herbs such as lavender and chamomile are gentle enough to use on the face. They can help to remove dead skin cells and impurities. These herbs can be used to make a facial scrub or added to facial steam to help open up pores and promote healthy circulation.

Moisturizers

In addition to their cleansing and exfoliating properties, alkaline herbs can be used as natural moisturizers. Herbs such as aloe vera and calendula contain soothing and hydrating properties that can help to soothe dry or irritated skin. These herbs can be used in various ways, including as an ingredient in a facial mask or an after-sun treatment.

Anti-Aging

Alkaline herbs such as rosemary and sage are also known for their anti-aging properties. These herbs contain antioxidants that can help to protect the skin from free radical damage and promote a youthful complexion. They can be used in various ways, including as an ingredient in a facial serum or added to facial steam to help improve skin elasticity.

Hair Care

Alkaline herbs can also be used for hair care. Herbs such as rosemary and lavender contain properties that can help to nourish and strengthen the hair. These herbs can be used in various ways, including as an ingredient in a hair rinse or added to a hair oil to promote healthy growth and shine.

Soothing Properties

Finally, many alkaline herbs contain soothing properties that help calm and soothe the skin. Herbs such as chamomile and lavender can be used in various ways, including as an ingredient in a facial mask or added to a bath to promote relaxation and reduce stress.

Chapter 3:
Sourcing Herbs

What Do You Mean By "Herb Sourcing"?

Sourcing herbs refers to obtaining or acquiring herbs for use in various culinary, medicinal, or cosmetic applications. This process includes selecting, procuring, transporting, and storing herbs. The quality and potency of herbs depend on several factors, including the conditions of their growth, harvesting methods, and the handling and processing they undergo during and after harvesting. Therefore, sourcing herbs involves finding the best sources and methods of obtaining high-quality herbs free from contaminants, adulterants, or other harmful substances.

Why Should You Source Your Own Herbs?

Herbs have been used for thousands of years for their medicinal, culinary, and aromatic properties. They are an essential part of many cultures and traditions. They are used in various products, from cosmetics and personal care items to food and drink. However, the quality and purity of herbs can vary greatly, depending on the source and processing methods used. This is why sourcing your own herbs is so important.

Ensuring Quality And Purity

One of the primary benefits of sourcing your own herbs is that you can ensure their quality and purity. When you grow your own herbs, you have control over how they are grown and processed. You can choose organic and sustainable methods free from chemicals and pesticides. You can harvest them at the right time to ensure the maximum potency and flavor.

Commercial herbs often contain fillers, additives, and preservatives to extend their shelf life and cut costs. These can reduce the potency and effectiveness of the herbs and may also cause adverse reactions in some people. By sourcing your own herbs, you can avoid these additives and enjoy the full benefits of the herbs in their purest form.

Connecting With Nature

Another benefit of sourcing your own herbs is that it allows you to connect with nature and the natural world. Gardening and growing herbs can be a meditative and calming practice that promotes mindfulness and self-care. It also encourages an appreciation for the natural world and the environment as you learn about the growing cycles of plants and the importance of soil health and biodiversity.

Growing herbs can be a great way to introduce children to the natural world and teach them the importance of sustainability and conservation. By involving them in planting, caring for, and harvesting herbs, you can help them develop an appreciation for the environment and an understanding of where their food and medicine come from.

Supporting Local And Sustainable Agriculture

Sourcing your own herbs also supports local and sustainable agriculture. Growing your own herbs reduces reliance on commercial herb suppliers, which often source herbs from other countries and use unsustainable farming practices. This can harm the environment and contribute to the exploitation of farmers and workers.

When you source your own herbs, you support local agriculture and small-scale farming, which is often more sustainable and eco-friendly. You can also choose to purchase seeds and plants from organic and fair-trade sources, which ensures that your herbs are grown in a way that supports the health of the planet and the people who grow them.

Cost-Effective Solution

Finally, sourcing your own herbs is a cost-effective way to enjoy the benefits of herbs. While herbs can be expensive to purchase in their dried or processed form, growing your own herbs can be a low-cost solution providing a constant supply of fresh and potent herbs.

Many herbs are easy to grow and require little maintenance, making them a great option for those with limited time, space, or resources. By growing your own herbs, you can also experiment with different varieties and flavors that may not be available at your local grocery store or herb supplier.

Factors To Consider When Sourcing A Herb

When it comes to sourcing herbs, several factors must be considered to ensure that they are high-quality, ethically sourced, and safe to use. Whether you are sourcing herbs for culinary, medicinal, or aromatic purposes, it's important to consider the following factors.

Growing and Harvesting Methods

The growing and harvesting methods used can significantly impact the quality and safety of the herbs. When sourcing herbs, it's important to consider the growing conditions, such as the soil quality, climate, and water source. It's also important to consider the harvesting methods used, such as handpicking or machine harvesting, as this can affect the quality and potency of the herbs.

Purity and Authenticity

Herbs can be vulnerable to adulteration, contamination, and misidentification, affecting their quality and safety. When sourcing herbs, it's important to ensure they are pure, authentic, and free from contaminants. This can be achieved by choosing a reliable and trusted source and checking for certifications, such as organic or fair-trade certifications.

Seasonal Availability

The availability of herbs can vary depending on the season and location. When sourcing herbs, it's important to consider the seasonal availability of the herbs and choose herbs that are in season and locally sourced. This can help ensure the herbs are fresh, potent, and sustainably grown.

Ethical and Sustainable Sourcing

Sourcing herbs ethically and sustainably is important for the environment and the people involved in the production process. When sourcing herbs, it's important to consider the ethical and sustainable practices of the suppliers and ensure that the herbs are grown and harvested using sustainable and eco-friendly methods. This can include choosing suppliers that use organic or fair-trade farming practices and support local agriculture.

Packaging and Storage

The way herbs are packaged and stored can have a significant impact on their quality and shelf life. When sourcing herbs, it's important to consider the packaging and storage methods used and choose herbs that have been packaged and stored in a way that preserves their quality and freshness. This can include choosing herbs that are stored in airtight containers and away from heat and light.

Different Sources Of Herbs To Consider

Herbs have been used for centuries for their medicinal, culinary, and aromatic properties. Sourcing herbs from a reliable and trusted source ensures their quality and potency. There are many different sources to consider when sourcing herbs, including local herb shops, online retailers, farmer markets, community-supported agriculture, herb gardens and farms, and wildcrafting.

Local Herb Shops

Local herb shops are a great source of high-quality herbs grown, harvested, and processed locally. These shops often work directly with local farmers and herb growers to source their products, ensuring that the herbs are fresh and of the highest quality. Local herb shops may also offer herbs and herbal products, including teas, tinctures, and essential oils.

Online Retailers

Online retailers are another popular source for herbs, especially for those who don't have access to a local herb shop or farmer's market. When choosing an online retailer, it's important to ensure that they have a good reputation and source their herbs from reliable and trusted suppliers. Online retailers may also offer a wider variety of herbs and herbal products than local shops and can often provide detailed information about the herbs they sell.

Farmer Markets

Farmer markets are an excellent source of fresh and locally-grown herbs. These markets offer various herbs and other produce, often sourced directly from the farmers who grow them. Buying herbs at a farmer's market allows you to speak directly with the farmers and learn more about their growing methods and harvesting practices. This can help ensure the herbs are fresh, high-quality, and grown sustainably.

Community Supported Agriculture

Community Supported Agriculture (CSA) is another great option for sourcing herbs. CSA programs allow consumers to buy a share in a local farm, which provides them with a regular supply of fresh, locally-grown produce, including herbs. CSA programs often offer a wide variety of herbs. They can provide information about the growing and harvesting methods used by the farmers.

Herb Gardens and Farms

Growing your own herbs in a home garden or visiting a local herb farm is an excellent way to source fresh, high-quality herbs. When growing your own herbs, you control the growing and harvesting methods, ensuring that the herbs are grown sustainably and free from harmful chemicals and pesticides. Visiting a local herb farm can also be a fun and educational experience, allowing you to learn more about the herbs and the farmers who grow them.

Wildcrafting

Wildcrafting is the practice of harvesting herbs and other plants from the wild. While this can be a sustainable and cost-effective way to source herbs, it's important to ensure you are harvesting them ethically and sustainably. When wildcrafting, it's important to follow best practices, such as harvesting only from healthy and abundant populations, leaving enough plants to ensure their survival, and avoiding harmful harvesting methods.

Tips For Sourcing Herbs

Herbs have been used for thousands of years for medicinal and culinary properties. With the growing interest in natural and holistic health, the demand for herbs is higher than ever. However, not all herbs are created equal, and it's important to source them properly to ensure they are of high quality and ethically sourced. Here are some tips for sourcing herbs:

Research Your Supplier

When sourcing herbs, it's important to research your supplier to ensure they are reputable and trustworthy. Look for suppliers with a strong reputation for providing high-quality herbs and are transparent about their sourcing practices. Check out their website, read reviews, and ask for recommendations from trusted sources.

Look for Certified Organic Herbs

Certified organic herbs are grown without synthetic fertilizers, pesticides, or herbicides. Look for suppliers that offer certified organic herbs to ensure they are free from harmful chemicals and toxins. Organic herbs are not only better for your health, but they arc also better for the environment and support sustainable agriculture.

Consider the Growing Conditions

The growing conditions of herbs can significantly impact their quality and potency. Look for suppliers that source their herbs from regions with ideal growing conditions. This may include specific soil types, climates, and altitudes. For example, ginseng grows best in the shade and requires a cool, moist environment.

Check for Freshness

Herbs lose their potency over time, so sourcing them from suppliers offering fresh herbs is important. Look for recently harvested herbs stored in a cool, dark, and dry place. Check the appearance and smell of the herbs to ensure they are fresh.

Ensure Ethical Sourcing

Many herbs are sourced from developing countries where labor laws are lax, and workers are often exploited. Look for suppliers that ensure ethical sourcing practices and fair wages for the workers involved in cultivating and harvesting the herbs. Consider purchasing herbs from suppliers that are certified by Fair Trade organizations.

Consider the Packaging

The packaging of herbs can also have an impact on their quality. Look for suppliers that package their herbs in airtight containers to prevent moisture and air exposure. This helps to maintain the freshness and potency of the herbs.

Check for Authenticity

Some herbs may be adulterated or mixed with other substances, affecting their quality and safety. Look for suppliers that test their herbs for authenticity and purity. This can involve DNA testing or chemical analysis to ensure that the herb is what it claims to be and doesn't contain harmful substances.

Consider the Harvesting Method

The harvesting method can also impact the quality of herbs. Some herbs are best harvested by hand to avoid damaging the plant and to ensure that the right parts of the plant are collected. Other herbs may be harvested by machine, but this can impact the quality of the herb. Look for suppliers that use the appropriate harvesting method for each herb.

Look for Whole Herbs

Whole herbs are typically more potent than processed or powdered herbs. When possible, look for suppliers that offer whole herbs that are minimally processed. This can help preserve the herb's natural oils, vitamins, and minerals.

Choose Local Herbs

Herbs grown and harvested locally may be fresher and of higher quality than herbs imported from other countries. Look for suppliers that offer locally grown herbs, or consider growing your own at home.

Chapter 4:
Harvesting And Growing Your Herbs

Harvesting and growing your own alkaline herbs is an excellent way to ensure you can access fresh, healthy herbs year-round. Whether you have a small garden or a large plot of land, growing your herbs is an easy and rewarding experience. This chapter will explore the different aspects of harvesting and growing your own alkaline herbs.

Choosing The Right Herb

Choosing the right alkaline herbs for growing is essential to creating a successful herb garden. With so many alkaline herbs available, knowing which ones to choose can be challenging. This section will explore the different factors to consider when selecting the right alkaline herbs for your garden.

Climate and Growing Conditions

The first factor to consider when choosing alkaline herbs for growing in your area's climate and growing conditions. Different herbs have varying requirements for sunlight, water, and soil type. For instance, Mediterranean herbs such as thyme, oregano, and rosemary thrive in hot, sunny, and dry conditions. At the same time, cilantro and parsley prefer cooler, shadier conditions with moist, well-drained soil. Therefore, it is important to research the growing conditions of different alkaline herbs before choosing which ones to plant in your garden.

Intended Use

Another crucial factor to consider when selecting the right alkaline herbs for growing is their intended use. Some herbs have distinct culinary or medicinal properties, making them ideal for particular uses. For example, basil and mint are commonly used in desserts and beverages. At the same time, rosemary and thyme are popular in savory dishes. Some herbs, such as chamomile, lavender, and echinacea, also have medicinal properties that can treat specific health conditions. Therefore, it is essential to research the different properties of different alkaline herbs to ensure that you choose the right ones for your intended use.

Ease of Growing and Maintenance

The ease of growing and maintaining different herbs is another crucial factor to consider when choosing alkaline herbs for growing. Some herbs are relatively easy to grow and require minimal care. In contrast, others are more challenging to cultivate and require more attention. For example, thyme, oregano, and sage are relatively low-maintenance herbs that require infrequent watering and minimal fertilizer, while basil and cilantro are more sensitive and require regular watering and more fertilization. Therefore, it is vital to consider your level of gardening experience and the amount of time and effort you are willing to dedicate to your herb garden when choosing which alkaline herbs to grow.

Availability and Cost

The availability and cost of different herbs are also essential when choosing alkaline herbs for growing. Some herbs may be more challenging to find or more expensive to purchase than others, making it more cost-effective to grow them yourself. For example, saffron is an expensive herb; growing it yourself can be more affordable. Additionally, by growing your own herbs, you can ensure that you always have fresh, healthy herbs on hand, which can be more convenient and cost-effective than purchasing herbs stored for a more extended period.

Planting And Growing Your Herbs

Once you have chosen the right alkaline herbs for your garden, the next step is to plant and grow them successfully. In this section, we will explore the steps and considerations to consider when planting and growing alkaline herbs.

Preparing the Soil

Preparing the soil is the first step in planting and growing alkaline herbs. Alkaline herbs thrive in well-draining, alkaline soil that is rich in nutrients. Therefore, testing your soil pH and adjusting it if necessary is important. You can use natural remedies such as wood ash or lime to raise the pH level of your soil or organic matter such as compost or manure to add nutrients and improve soil texture. Before planting, ensure that the soil is thoroughly mixed and aerated and that any weeds or debris are removed.

Choosing the Right Location

The location of your herb garden is also a critical factor to consider when planting and growing alkaline herbs. Most herbs require full sun, at least six hours of direct sunlight daily, and a warm, sheltered location. However, some herbs like cilantro and parsley prefer partial shade, particularly in hotter climates. Ensure your chosen location is not too windy or exposed, and the soil drains well to prevent waterlogging and root rot.

Planting and Care

Once you have prepared the soil and chosen the right location, it is time to plant your alkaline herbs. Begin by digging a hole slightly larger than the root ball of your herb and adding a layer of organic matter or compost to the bottom of the hole. Gently place the herb in the hole and backfill it with soil, ensuring that the herb is planted at the same depth as it was in its original container. Water the herb thoroughly after planting. Water it regularly to ensure the soil remains moist but not waterlogged.

In addition to watering, it is also important to fertilize your alkaline herbs regularly to promote healthy growth and prevent nutrient deficiencies. Organic fertilizers such as compost tea or fish emulsion are ideal for herbs and provide essential nutrients without causing soil imbalance. Additionally, prune your herbs regularly to encourage bushy growth and prevent overcrowding.

Harvesting Your Herbs

Harvesting your alkaline herbs is a crucial step in growing and using them. Once your herbs are mature, it is important to harvest them at the right time and in the right way to ensure maximum flavor and potency. In this section, we will explore the steps and considerations to remember when harvesting alkaline herbs.

Timing

Timing is critical when it comes to harvesting your alkaline herbs. Most herbs are at their peak flavor and potency just before they flower. For example, basil is best harvested before it flowers to ensure the best flavor, while lavender is best harvested when the flowers are fully open. Monitoring your herbs regularly and harvesting them when they are young and tender for the best results is important.

Tools

The tools you use for harvesting your herbs can also impact their flavor and quality. Use clean, sharp scissors or pruning shears to harvest the herbs, and do not damage the plant.

Using dull or dirty tools can introduce bacteria or disease to the plant, affecting its health and flavor.

Method

There are different methods for harvesting your alkaline herbs, depending on the type of herb and how you plan to use it. For leafy herbs such as basil, parsley, and mint, you can snip off individual leaves or cut back the entire plant to encourage bushy growth. For herbs with woody stems, such as thyme and rosemary, you can trim off the top few inches of the stem or cut back the entire plant to promote new growth.

Drying And Storing Your Herbs

Drying and storing alkaline herbs is essential to herb harvesting and preservation. Proper drying and storage help maintain the freshness of the herbs and increase their shelf life, making them available for use over a more extended period. Here are some guidelines to help you dry and store your alkaline herbs.

Harvesting the Herbs

Before you start drying and storing your herbs, it is important to properly harvest them. Harvesting your herbs at the right time is crucial for the potency and flavor of the herbs. The best time to harvest your herbs is in the morning after the dew has dried but before the sun is too hot. Always harvest only healthy herbs, avoiding any plants showing signs of disease or insect infestation.

Drying the Herbs

Drying is the most common method of preserving herbs. It is essential to dry herbs thoroughly to avoid mold or other forms of spoilage. There are several ways to dry herbs, including air-drying, oven-drying, and dehydrating. Air-drying is the easiest and most economical method of drying herbs, requiring no special equipment. To air-dry your herbs, tie the stems together and hang them upside down in a warm, dry, and well-ventilated area. Ensure to keep the herbs away from direct sunlight, which can cause them to lose their potency.

Oven drying is a faster method of drying herbs but requires more attention to prevent scorching. To oven-dry, your herbs, place them on a baking sheet and bake them at a low temperature of about 100 to 150 degrees Fahrenheit for about 2 to 4 hours. Dehydrating is another effective method of drying herbs that requires a dehydrator. Follow the instructions of your dehydrator to ensure your herbs are thoroughly dried.

Storing the Herbs

After drying, it is crucial to store your herbs properly to maintain their potency and flavor. Herbs should be stored in a cool, dry, and dark place to avoid light and moisture, which can cause the herbs to lose their potency and spoil. Glass jars with tight-fitting lids are the best containers for storing herbs, as they help maintain the herbs' freshness and aroma.

Labeling and Dating the Herbs

Proper labeling and dating of your herbs are essential to ensure you use them before they lose their potency. Label your jars with the herb's name and the date you harvested and dried them. Use a permanent marker to avoid smudging or fading. Herbs typically lose their potency after about a year, so using them within that time is essential.

Chapter 5:
Preparing The Herbs For Usage And Appropriate Dosage

Infusions And Decoctions

What are Infusions and Decoctions? Infusions and decoctions are two methods of preparing herbal teas. Infusions are made by pouring boiling water over the herbs and letting them steep for a certain period. They are commonly used for delicate plant parts like leaves, flowers, and soft stems. Decoctions, conversely, are made by simmering the herbs in boiling water for a longer period. They are commonly used for hard plant parts like roots, bark, and seeds.

How to Use Infusions and Decoctions for Alkaline Herbs Alkaline herbs can be prepared using infusions and decoctions. The method used will depend on the specific herb and the plant part being used. Infusions are best suited for alkaline herbs with delicate plant parts like leaves. At the same time, decoctions are best for alkaline herbs with harder plant parts like roots and bark.

Step-by-Step Guide for Making an Infusion Here's how to make an infusion using alkaline herbs:

1. Bring water to a boil in a pot or kettle.

2. Measure out one tablespoon of dried herbs per cup of water.

3. Place the herbs in a tea strainer or tea ball.

4. Place the tea strainer or tea ball into a cup or teapot.

5. Pour the boiling water over the herbs.

6. Cover the cup or teapot with a lid or plate to keep the steam in.

7. Let the herbs steep for 10-15 minutes or longer for a stronger infusion.

8. Remove the tea strainer or tea ball from the cup or teapot.

9. Drink the infusion while it is still warm.

Step-by-Step Guide for Making a Decoction Here's how to make a decoction using alkaline herbs:

1. Bring water to a boil in a pot or kettle.

2. Measure out one tablespoon of dried herbs per cup of water.

3. Place the herbs in the pot of boiling water.

4. Reduce the heat to low and let the herbs simmer for 20-30 minutes or longer for a stronger decoction.

5. Remove the pot from the heat.

6. Strain the liquid into a cup or container using a strainer or cheesecloth.

7. Drink the decoction while it is still warm.

Tinctures And Extracts

What are Tinctures and Extracts? Tinctures and extracts are two methods of preparing herbal remedies. They are made by soaking the herbs in alcohol or a solvent for a certain period to extract the active ingredients. Tinctures are made using alcohol and water, while extracts can be made using alcohol, water, or glycerin. Tinctures are often used for faster-acting and more potent remedies. In contrast, extracts are used for more mild and more gentle remedies.

How to Use Tinctures and Extracts for Alkaline Herbs Alkaline herbs can be prepared using tinctures and extracts. The type of method used will depend on the specific herb and the desired potency of the remedy. Tinctures are best suited for alkaline herbs with high concentrations of essential oils. In contrast, extracts are best suited for alkaline herbs with low concentrations of essential oils.

Step-by-Step Guide for Making a Tincture Here's how to make a tincture using alkaline herbs:

1. Choose the herb you want to use and gather the necessary equipment, including a glass jar with a tight-fitting lid, alcohol (at least 40% proof), and a scale.

2. Weigh the dried herb and add it to the glass jar.

3. Pour enough alcohol over the herb to cover it completely.

4. Close the lid tightly and shake the jar vigorously.

5. Store the jar in a cool, dark place for at least 4-6 weeks, shaking it daily.

6. After 4-6 weeks, strain the liquid using a cheesecloth or strainer.

7. Store the tincture in a dark bottle with a dropper for easy use.

Step-by-Step Guide for Making an Extract Here's how to make an extract using alkaline herbs:

1. Choose the herb you want to use and gather the necessary equipment, including a glass jar with a tight-fitting lid, alcohol or glycerin, and a scale.

2. Weigh the dried herb and add it to the glass jar.

3. Pour enough alcohol or glycerin over the herb to cover it completely.

4. Close the lid tightly and shake the jar vigorously.

5. Store the jar in a cool, dark place for at least 4-6 weeks, shaking it daily.

6. After 4-6 weeks, strain the liquid using a cheesecloth or strainer.

7. Store the extract in a dark bottle with a dropper for easy use.

Capsules And Tablets

Capsules and tablets are two convenient methods used to consume alkaline herbs. They are an easy way to consume herbs without brewing tea or creating tinctures or extracts. In this guide, we will discuss what capsules and tablets are, how they can be used to prepare alkaline herbs, and provide a step-by-step guide on how to do it.

What are Capsules and Tablets? Capsules and tablets are oral dosage forms used to deliver medication or supplements to the body. Capsules are small, cylindrical-shaped containers filled with powdered or liquid substances. At the same time, tablets are small, solid, and often coated in a substance to make them easier to swallow.

How to Use Capsules and Tablets for Alkaline Herbs Alkaline herbs can be prepared using capsules and tablets. The type of method used will depend on the specific herb and the desired potency of the remedy. Capsules are best suited for alkaline herbs with a strong taste or smell. In contrast, tablets are best suited for alkaline herbs with more active ingredients.

Step-by-Step Guide for Making Capsules Here's how to make capsules using alkaline herbs:

1. Choose the herb you want to use and gather the necessary equipment, including a capsule machine, empty capsules, and a scale.

2. Weigh the dried herb and place it in a clean, dry bowl.

3. Open the empty capsules and separate the two halves.

4. Fill the bottom half of the capsule with the herb using the capsule machine.

5. Close the capsule by pressing the top half onto the bottom using the capsule machine.

6. Repeat the process until you have the desired number of capsules.

7. Store the capsules in a clean, dry container in a cool, dark place.

Step-by-Step Guide for Making Tablets Here's how to make tablets using alkaline herbs:

1. Choose the herb you want to use and gather the necessary equipment, including a tablet press, tablet mold, and a scale.

2. Weigh the dried herb and place it in a clean, dry bowl.

3. Mix the herb with a binding agent such as starch or gum arabic.

4. Press the mixture into the tablet mold using the tablet press.

5. Remove the tablet from the mold and let it dry in a cool, dry place.

6. Repeat the process until you have the desired number of tablets.

7. Store the tablets in a clean, dry container in a cool, dark place.

Poultices And Compresses

What are Poultices and Compresses? A poultice is a moist, warm mixture of herbs applied to the skin to treat various ailments. It can be made using fresh or dried herbs and is typically placed on the skin and covered with a cloth or bandage. A compress is a similar method but is typically cold and can be used to reduce inflammation or swelling.

How to Use Poultices and Compresses for Alkaline Herbs Alkaline herbs can prepare and compresses to treat various health conditions. The type of herb used will depend on the specific condition being treated. Poultices and compresses are best used for external conditions such as skin irritations, bruises, muscle pain, and inflammation.

Step-by-Step Guide for Making a Poultice Here's how to make a poultice using alkaline herbs:

1. Choose the herb you want to use and gather the necessary equipment, including a mortar and pestle, a bowl, and a cloth or bandage.

2. Crush the herb in the mortar and pestle until it is a fine powder or paste.

3. Mix the herb with enough water to make a thick, moist paste.

4. Apply the paste to the affected area of the skin.

5. Cover the paste with a clean cloth or bandage.

6. Leave the poultice on for at least 20 minutes or as long as needed.

7. Remove the poultice and discard any leftover paste.

Step-by-Step Guide for Making a Compress Here's how to make a compress using alkaline herbs:

1. Choose the herb you want to use and gather the necessary equipment, including a bowl, a clean cloth, and a towel.

2. Brew a strong tea using the herb and hot water.

3. Soak the cloth in the tea.

4. Apply the cloth to the affected area of the skin.

5. Cover the cloth with a towel to keep it in place.

6. Leave the compress on for at least 20 minutes or as long as needed.

7. Remove the compress and discard any leftover tea.

Salves And Cream

What are Salves and Creams? Salves and creams are semi-solid mixtures of oils and waxes infused with herbs. They are used topically to treat skin conditions such as dryness, itching, and inflammation. Salves are thicker and more concentrated than creams and are ideal for use on areas of the body that are prone to dryness, such as the hands and feet.

How to Use Salves and Creams for Alkaline Herbs Alkaline herbs can prepare salves and creams to treat various skin conditions. The type of herb used will depend on the specific condition being treated. Salves and creams are best used for external conditions such as dry skin, eczema, and minor wounds.

Step-by-Step Guide for Making a Salve Here's how to make a salve using alkaline herbs:

1. Choose the herb you want to use and gather the necessary equipment, including a double boiler, a glass jar, a strainer, a cheesecloth, and a small tin or jar to store the finished salve.

2. Grind the herb into a fine powder using a mortar, pestle, or coffee grinder.

3. Place the powdered herb into the glass jar.

4. Heat the oil and beeswax in the double boiler until the wax is melted.

5. Pour the melted oil and wax mixture into the glass jar with the herb.

6. Stir the mixture well and let it steep for several hours or overnight.

7. Strain the mixture through a cheesecloth to remove any plant material.

8. Pour the strained mixture into a small tin or jar.

9. Allow the salve to cool and harden before using.

Step-by-Step Guide for Making a Cream Here's how to make a cream using alkaline herbs:

1. Choose the herb you want to use and gather the necessary equipment, including a double boiler, a glass jar, a strainer, a cheesecloth, and a small jar to store the finished cream.

2. Grind the herb into a fine powder using a mortar, pestle, or coffee grinder.

3. Heat the oil and beeswax in the double boiler until the wax is melted.

4. Pour the melted oil and wax mixture into the glass jar with the herb.

5. Stir the mixture well and let it steep for several hours or overnight.

6. Strain the mixture through a cheesecloth to remove any plant material.

7. Add a small amount of water or aloe vera gel to the strained mixture and stir well.

8. Pour the cream into a small jar.

9. Allow the cream to cool and thicken before using.

What To Consider When Choosing A Method?

Choosing a method for preparing alkaline herbs can depend on several factors, including the specific herb you are using, the intended use of the herb, and your personal preferences. Here are some things to consider when selecting a preparation method for your alkaline herbs:

1. Type of herb: Different herbs may be more effective when prepared differently. For example, some herbs are better extracted with alcohol, while others are better extracted with water.

2. Intended use: The preparation method can also depend on the intended use of the herb. For example, if you use an herb to treat a skin condition, you may prefer a topical preparation like a salve or cream. You may prefer tea or tincture if you use an herb for digestive issues.

3. Convenience: Some preparation methods may be more convenient than others. For example, capsules and tablets are easy to take on the go, while making a decoction or infusion can take some time and effort.
4. Personal preference: Some people may prefer one preparation method over another due to personal preference or taste. For example, some people may prefer the taste of tea over a tincture or the convenience of a capsule over tea.
5. Safety: It's important to consider the safety of the preparation method, as some methods can be riskier than others. For example, making a tincture with high-proof alcohol can be dangerous if safety precautions are not taken.

Ultimately, the method of preparing alkaline herbs will depend on the specific herb and the intended use, as well as personal preference and safety considerations. It's important to do research and consult with a healthcare professional before using any new herbs or herbal preparations.

Chapter 6:
Propretés of Most Common Herbs

Arnica

Arnica, a herb with a rich history in medicinal practices, predominantly hails from Europe, especially the mountainous terrains of the Alps. However, its prominence isn't limited to Europe; arnica's therapeutic virtues have led to its cultivation across diverse territories including North America and Asia. This sunflower family member stands out for its impressive anti-inflammatory and pain-alleviating attributes. It's often the first choice for treating ailments like bruises, sprains, and conditions like osteoarthritis and rheumatoid arthritis.

One of the lesser-known qualities of arnica is its antimicrobial capabilities. These properties not only guard against infections but also play a pivotal role in the healing process. Additionally, arnica has the unique ability to encourage blood flow to areas of injury or inflammation, which in turn can minimize swelling and expedite the recovery process.

Dr. Sebi, a renowned herbalist, has always advocated for harnessing the power of natural herbs and plants for health betterment. Arnica holds a special place in Dr. Sebi's diet, primarily due to its bounty of phytochemicals that contribute to its anti-inflammatory and pain-relieving prowess. These components not only promote health but also act as a shield against certain chronic diseases.

When it comes to the alkaline diet, arnica's inherent alkalizing characteristics make it a valuable addition. Its elevated pH profile complements meals crafted to foster body alkalinity. Beyond this, arnica is also known to have a calming influence on the digestive system, mitigating inflammation and bolstering digestive wellness.

Nevertheless, as with many potent herbs, caution is essential. While arnica is a treasure trove of benefits when applied topically in the form of creams or gels, ingesting it, especially in excessive amounts, can be hazardous due to its internal toxicity.

In essence, while arnica's medicinal prominence spanning centuries is commendable, and its fit in diets like Dr. Sebi's or the alkaline regime is notable, it's crucial to employ it wisely, primarily for external applications. This approach ensures that one can reap its benefits for holistic health without inadvertently exposing oneself to risks.

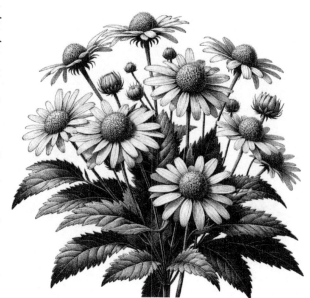

Batana

Hailing from the lush rainforests of Central America, especially Honduras, Panama, and Costa Rica, Batana, commonly known as Ojon, is not just an ordinary plant. Indigenous communities, particularly the Miskito people of Honduras and Nicaragua, have cherished it for its multifaceted benefits for ages. Its use extends far beyond just medicinal, serving also as a staple food source and even as a protective shield against bothersome insects.

Diving deeper into its traditional significance, the oil from Batana's nuts stands out. Indigenous communities have leveraged its potent properties to counter a myriad of health concerns, from addressing digestive quandaries to soothing skin afflictions. Its versatility even makes it a formidable natural insect repellent, safeguarding against parasitic woes.

With the beauty industry's ever-growing penchant for natural and effective ingredients, it's no surprise that Batana oil has earned a revered spot. It's a treasure trove of fatty acids, especially oleic acid, which imparts a deep moisturizing effect for both skin and hair. The antioxidant-rich nature of the oil also plays a pivotal role in shielding skin from the bane of environmental aggressors, such as pollutants and harmful UV rays. The anti-inflammatory attributes further amplify its allure, potentially easing skin irritations and redness.

And that's not all. The richness of vitamin E in Batana oil, complemented by an array of nutrients like vitamin A, iron, and calcium, makes it an impeccable choice for radiant skin and lustrous hair. Vitamin E, known for its robust antioxidant properties, offers dual benefits: defending skin from oxidative threats and possibly curbing the onset of age-related signs.

42

Shifting the focus to dietary considerations, the Dr. Sebi Diet accentuates the virtues of alkaline-forming, plant-based edibles. Batana, with its alkaline orientation and nutrient richness, seamlessly fits into this dietary philosophy. It not only balances the body's pH spectrum but also offers a nutrient-packed alternative to animal-derived oils, which are often criticized for their saturated fat content.

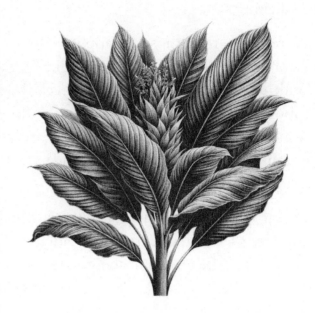

In summation, Batana is more than just a plant; it's a legacy of centuries, interweaving medicinal, culinary, and cosmetic narratives. As an emblem of health and wellness, it harmoniously blends into holistic, plant-centric diets, making it an invaluable asset for those committed to a rejuvenated health journey. Whether as a culinary delight, a guardian against pests, or a beauty elixir, Batana emerges as an indispensable ally.

Bladderwrack

Growing along the rocky contours of the Atlantic and Pacific Oceans, Bladderwrack, also recognized as Fucus vesiculosus, isn't just another seaweed. It's been a beacon of holistic health and traditional medicine for ages, especially revered in areas like Ireland, Scotland, Wales, and France's Brittany coast.

With its deep green tendrils, Bladderwrack is more than a mere marine plant. It's a reservoir of myriad health benefits, making it a standout in the realm of natural remedies. One of its crowning achievements lies in its rich iodine content. Iodine is the thyroid gland's best friend, helping to maintain its optimal function. A dip in iodine levels can thrust the body into the lull of hypothyroidism, leading to a cascade of issues like persistent fatigue, unexpected weight gain, and even parched skin.

But Bladderwrack's prowess doesn't stop there. Within its composition lies fucoidan, a compound that boasts significant anti-inflammatory capabilities. And given how inflammation often walks hand-in-hand with ailments like arthritis and heart conditions, it's no surprise that Bladderwrack is cherished. Its antioxidative properties, fueled by its ability to fend off menacing free radicals, further solidify its standing. Such free radicals have been implicated in a slew of health challenges, from heart conditions to the ravages of Alzheimer's.

Moreover, for those grappling with digestive inconsistencies, Bladderwrack might be the answer. With its high fiber quotient, it paves the way for a robust digestive system, ensuring things move smoothly. And not to be overlooked are its potential immune-enhancing traits, serving as a guardian against infections.

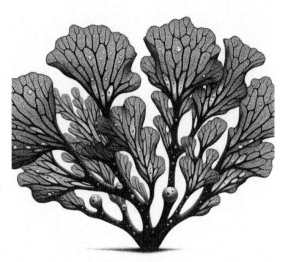

Diving into its alkaline attributes, Bladderwrack emerges as a veritable treasure. Laden with minerals like calcium, magnesium, and potassium, it functions as an alkalinity champion, helping neutralize excessive body acidity. This not only fosters a hospitable environment for overall health but also wards off challenges like acid reflux and joint discomfort.

Within the framework of the Dr. Sebi Diet, Bladderwrack's importance becomes even clearer. Dr. Sebi, an advocate for alkaline-centric nutrition, perceived such foods as the bedrock of disease prevention. Given Bladderwrack's alkaline edge and multifaceted benefits, it slots perfectly into this dietary philosophy.

In essence, Bladderwrack, a time-tested gem from traditional medicine, is an invaluable ally for holistic well-being. Its alignment with the Dr. Sebi Diet underscores its potential in paving the way for a healthier life. However, as with any potent herb, it's wise to seek guidance from healthcare professionals before making it a staple in one's regimen.

Blessed Thistle

Hailing from the sunny stretches of the Mediterranean, blessed thistle, often referred to as holy thistle, is a herbal marvel with deep roots in natural medicine. In our exploration today, we'll delve into the rich history and myriad benefits of this revered herb and shed light on its significance in the context of the Dr. Sebi and alkaline diets.

Blessed thistle, scientifically termed Cnicus benedictus, is no foreigner to North America. Thanks to the early settlers, this Mediterranean native found its way across the seas. A relative of the milk thistle and artichoke, blessed thistle proudly stands as an annual plant, stretching up to three feet, adorned with prickly leaves and striking yellow blooms. It thrives in the parched, stony terrains scattered across Europe, Asia, and Africa.

Throughout the annals of history, blessed thistle has carved a niche for itself as a potent remedy for a spectrum of ailments. Whether it's the unease of digestive troubles, a dwindling appetite, or the complexities of hormonal imbalances, this herb has been a trusted ally. New mothers have also turned to it as a natural galactagogue, stimulating breast milk production. While some studies hint at its potential antiviral and anticancer prowess, the scientific world awaits more concrete evidence.

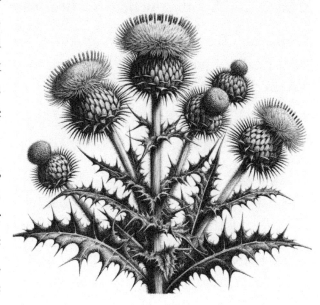

Peeling back the layers of this herbal wonder, one discovers a treasure trove of compounds. Among them, sesquiterpene lactones shine for their anti-inflammatory and antioxidative properties. The herb's tannin content, meanwhile, lends a hand in quelling digestive inflammation and ensuring smooth digestive processes.

But where does blessed thistle fit in the Dr. Sebi and alkaline diet landscapes? Both these dietary philosophies champion the virtues of unprocessed, natural foods that usher in a harmonious pH equilibrium in the body. Blessed thistle, with its inherent alkaline nature, emerges as a hero in neutralizing the body's excessive acidity. And in a world where acid-loaded diets wreak havoc, manifesting as inflammation, digestive challenges, and even chronic ailments, such herbs are nothing short of saviors.

The benefits of blessed thistle are manifold, extending from enhanced digestion to curbing inflammation. For those navigating the path of the Dr. Sebi or alkaline diets, this herb is a shining beacon. Its acid-neutralizing abilities combined with its myriad health benefits render it a prized addition to any health-conscious individual's dietary regimen.

Blue Vervain

Nestled in the verdant expanses of North America lies the Blue Vervain, a perennial herb scientifically christened Verbena hastata. A cherished member of the Verbenaceae family, this plant's roots trace back to ancient medicinal practices, particularly in the continent's eastern expanses.

A genuine product of North America, Blue Vervain was revered by the indigenous Native American tribes who recognized and harnessed its potent medicinal prowess. This herb's unmistakable presence can be spotted adorning meadows, fields, and roadsides in the United States' eastern territories, with states such as Florida, Illinois, Texas, and New York being notable hotspots. Its reach, however, isn't confined to the U.S. alone - parts of Canada, Mexico, and South America too, bear witness to its growth.

Medicinal Treasury: Blue Vervain is a veritable goldmine of therapeutic properties. Historically, it has been celebrated for its unmatched ability to soothe and pacify the nervous system. Let's journey through some of its myriad benefits:

- Mental Well-being: Entrusted as a guardian of mental health, Blue Vervain stands as a bulwark against anxiety, stress, and nervousness, all thanks to its tranquilizing virtues.

- Sleep's Best Friend: For those tormented by insomnia, Blue Vervain emerges as a beacon of hope, inviting restful and rejuvenating sleep.

- Digestive Aid: This herb is also hailed as a digestive tonic, battling constipation and spurring a robust appetite.

- Respiratory Relief: Breathing troubles, be it asthma or persistent coughs, find a worthy adversary in Blue Vervain due to its expectorant qualities.

- Women's Ally: A special mention for its role in women's health. Blue Vervain has been entrusted to harmonize menstrual cycles and alleviate associated cramps.

Dr. Sebi, a venerated herbalist and natural healer, constructed the Dr. Sebi Diet around a core tenet: diseases find fertile ground in acidic environments. Central to this dietary regimen is the consumption of alkaline foods while sidelining their acidic counterparts. And in this alkaline universe, Blue Vervain shines brightly. Its believed alkaline-forming attributes make it a coveted herb in Dr. Sebi's list. Similarly, those who advocate for the Alkaline Diet also embrace Blue Vervain, given its alkaline nature.

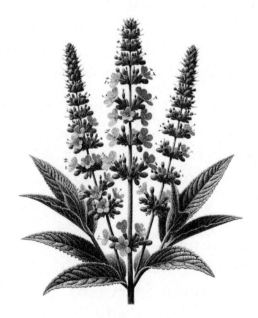

In the vast tapestry of natural medicine, Blue Vervain occupies a position of pride. Whether you're an adherent of the Dr. Sebi diet, an Alkaline diet enthusiast, or simply someone looking to embrace nature's healing touch, Blue Vervain stands ready to enrich your health journey.

Bromide Plus

Bromide Plus is an herbal supplement created by the late Dr. Sebi, a naturalist and healer who believed a plant-based diet could cure various health conditions. Bromide Plus combines several herbs, including Bladderwrack, Sea moss, and Burdock root. It is believed to have many health benefits, particularly for those following a Dr. Sebi Diet.

Bladderwrack is a seaweed rich in iodine and other minerals, including calcium, magnesium, and potassium. Sea moss is also a type of seaweed high in minerals and other nutrients, including vitamins A, C, E, and K. Burdock root is a natural diuretic believed to help detoxify the body and improve digestion.

In terms of its suitability for a Dr. Sebi Diet, Bromide Plus is considered to be an alkaline-forming supplement. The Dr. Sebi Diet is a plant-based diet that emphasizes the consumption of whole, natural foods that are alkaline-forming and have a high nutrient content. The goal of the diet is to promote optimal health and prevent disease by maintaining a balanced pH level in the body.

Bromide Plus is believed to have several potential health benefits. It is thought to help support the immune system, improve digestion and nutrient absorption, and promote healthy skin, hair, and nails. It is also believed to have a calming effect on the body, reducing anxiety and promoting restful sleep.

Bromide Plus is typically consumed as a powder or capsule; the appropriate dosage can vary depending on an individual's needs and health status. It is important to consult with a healthcare professional before incorporating Bromide Plus into your diet to determine the appropriate dosage and ensure it is safe for you.

Burdock Root

Burdock Root, also known as Arctium lappa, is a biennial plant that belongs to the Asteraceae family. It is native to Europe and Asia but is now naturalized in North America and other parts of the world. Burdock Root has been used for centuries in traditional medicine for its various health benefits.

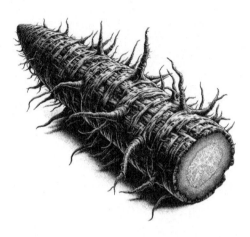

Origins and Distribution: The ancient Greeks and Romans used Burdock Root in traditional Chinese medicine for thousands of years for its medicinal properties. It is now widely cultivated in different parts of the world, including Europe, Asia, and North America. Burdock Root is commonly found in fields, meadows, and along roadsides.

Benefits and Uses: Burdock Root has numerous health benefits and has been used in traditional medicine to treat various ailments. Some of the benefits and uses of this herb include:

1. Skin Health: Burdock Root is known to improve skin health by treating various skin conditions such as eczema, psoriasis, and acne. It has antibacterial and anti-inflammatory properties that help treat these conditions.

2. Liver Health: Burdock Root is believed to improve liver function by detoxifying the liver and promoting the excretion of toxins from the body.

3. Digestive Health: Burdock Root stimulates digestion, relieves constipation, and promotes a healthy appetite.

4. Blood Sugar Management: Burdock root is believed to lower blood sugar levels and improve insulin sensitivity, making it useful for managing diabetes.

5. Anti-inflammatory Properties: Burdock Root has anti-inflammatory properties that make it useful in treating various inflammatory conditions such as arthritis and gout.

Dr. Sebi Diet and Alkaline Diet: Burdock Root is recommended for the Dr. Sebi Diet, which is based on the principle of consuming alkaline foods and avoiding acidic foods. The Dr. Sebi Diet emphasizes consuming plant-based foods rich in nutrients and minerals. Burdock Root is considered alkaline-forming in the body, making it a suitable addition to this diet.

Similarly, Burdock Root is also recommended for the Alkaline Diet, which is based on the principle of consuming alkaline foods and avoiding acidic foods. The Alkaline Diet promotes overall health and well-being by maintaining the body's pH. Burdock Root is considered to be an alkaline herb, making it a suitable addition to this diet.

Cascara Sagrada

In the dense forests of the Pacific Northwest region of North America, a particular tree stands with a rich history of medicinal use — Cascara Sagrada. Scientifically recognized as Rhamnus purshiana, it belongs to the buckthorn family and has found its way into many traditional medicine practices.

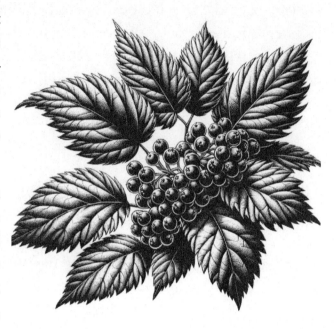

Origins and Distribution: Cascara Sagrada is a deciduous tree, which, though modest in size — growing up to 20 meters — has a profound impact in the world of traditional medicine. Its roots trace back to the Pacific Northwest regions, such as British Columbia, Washington, and Oregon. Ideally, the tree flourishes in damp habitats, which explains its penchant for riverbanks, valleys, and lush forests.

The Cascade of Benefits: This tree isn't just known for its sturdy bark and vast reach; its medicinal contributions are of significant note. Here are some of the highlights:

- Battle Against Constipation: The bark of Cascara Sagrada emerges as a champion for those grappling with constipation. Its natural laxative properties ensure regular bowel movements.

- Digestive Dynamism: In the grand machinery of digestion, Cascara Sagrada acts as a catalyst. It fosters the secretion of digestive enzymes and amplifies the health of the digestive system.

- Liver's Ally: Toxins often plague the liver, and Cascara Sagrada assists in their expulsion, ensuring the liver functions at its prime.

- Anti-inflammatory Advocate: Inflammation meets its nemesis in Cascara Sagrada. Conditions such as arthritis can potentially find relief through its anti-inflammatory properties.

Dietary Discourse: While Cascara Sagrada's attributes are commendable, it doesn't find favor in certain dietary realms, such as the Dr. Sebi Diet and the Alkaline Diet. Both these diets revolve around the axis of alkalinity. Cascara Sagrada, however, leans towards acidity. Therefore, within these dietary frameworks, this herb doesn't quite fit in. The philosophy of both diets prioritizes alkaline foods and pushes acidic ones to the periphery. Given Cascara Sagrada's acidic nature, it stands as an outlier.

Cascara Sagrada, with its spectrum of benefits, exemplifies nature's power to heal. However, its integration into one's diet or medicinal routine should be approached with discernment, especially when considering specific dietary frameworks. Always remember that natural doesn't always mean universally suitable, and it's wise to tread with knowledge and, if needed, professional advice.

Chaparral

Chaparral, also known as Larrea tridentata, is a small, evergreen shrub native to the southwestern region of the United States and the northern region of Mexico. It has been used for centuries in traditional medicine for its antioxidant, antimicrobial, and anti-inflammatory properties.

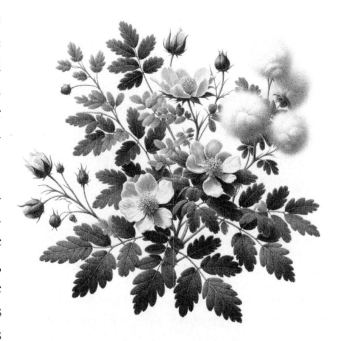

Origins and Distribution: Chaparral is a perennial shrub that grows up to 4 meters tall. It is native to the southwestern region of the United States, including California, Arizona, New Mexico, and Texas, as well as the northern region of Mexico. The shrub is commonly found in desert areas. It has adapted to the arid climate by developing thick leaves that prevent water loss.

Benefits and Uses: Chaparral has a long history of use in traditional medicine for its antioxidant, antimicrobial, and anti-inflammatory properties. Some of the benefits and uses of this herb include:

1. Antioxidant Properties: Chaparral is rich in antioxidants, which protect the body from damage caused by free radicals.

2. Anti-inflammatory Properties: Chaparral has anti-inflammatory properties that make it useful in treating various inflammatory conditions such as arthritis.

3. Antimicrobial Properties: Chaparral has antimicrobial properties that make it useful in treating various bacterial and fungal infections.

4. Skin Health: Chaparral is believed to promote skin health by reducing inflammation and protecting against damage caused by UV radiation.

Dr. Sebi Diet and Alkaline Diet: Chaparral is not recommended for the Dr. Sebi Diet or the Alkaline Diet. The Dr. Sebi Diet is based on the principle of consuming foods that are alkaline and avoiding foods that are acidic. Chaparral is considered an acidic herb, making it unsuitable for this diet.

Similarly, Chaparral is also not recommended for the Alkaline Diet, which is based on the principle of consuming alkaline foods and avoiding acidic foods. The Alkaline Diet is believed to promote overall health and well-being by maintaining the body's pH level. Chaparral is considered to be an acidic herb, making it unsuitable for this diet.

It is important to note that Chaparral has been associated with liver toxicity and banned in some countries for this reason. While it has numerous health benefits, it is important to use it under the guidance of a healthcare professional.

Cocolmeca

Cocolmeca, also known as Smilax ornata, is a perennial vine native to Central and South America. It has been used for centuries in traditional medicine for its anti-inflammatory and detoxifying properties.

Origins and Distribution: Cocolmeca is a vine that grows up to 6 meters long and is native to Central and South America. It is commonly found in tropical and subtropical regions, including Mexico, Costa Rica, and Colombia. The vine has thorny stems and produces small, fragrant flowers that develop into red or black berries.

Benefits and Uses: Cocolmeca has a long history of use in traditional medicine for its anti-inflammatory and detoxifying properties. Some of the benefits and uses of this herb include:

1. Anti-inflammatory Properties: Cocolmeca has anti-inflammatory properties that make it useful in treating various inflammatory conditions such as arthritis, gout, and joint pain.

2. Detoxifying Properties: Cocolmeca is believed to have detoxifying properties that can help remove toxins from the body and promote overall health.

3. Digestive Health: Cocolmeca is believed to promote digestive health by reducing inflammation in the digestive tract and improving nutrient absorption.

4. Skin Health: Cocolmeca is believed to promote skin health by reducing inflammation and promoting the healing of wounds and skin conditions.

Dr. Sebi Diet and Alkaline Diet: Cocolmeca is recommended for the Dr. Sebi Diet, which is based on the principle of consuming alkaline foods and avoiding acidic foods. Cocolmeca is considered to be an alkaline herb, making it suitable for this diet.

Similarly, Cocolmeca is also recommended for the Alkaline Diet, which is based on the principle of consuming alkaline foods and avoiding acidic foods. The Alkaline Diet promotes overall health and well-being by maintaining the body's pH. Cocolmeca is considered to be an alkaline herb, making it suitable for this diet.

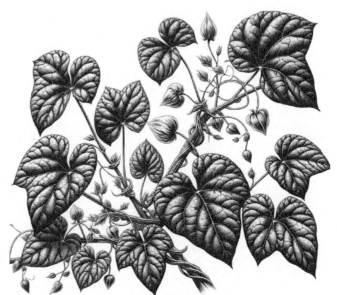

In addition to its use in traditional medicine, Cocolmeca has also been studied for its potential as a natural remedy for various health conditions. Research has suggested that the herb may be useful in treating diabetes, high blood pressure, and kidney stones. However, more research is needed to fully understand the health benefits of Cocolmeca and potential side effects.

Contribo

In the lush canopy of the Amazon Rainforest, a herb has made its mark through the annals of time: Contribo. Known by the names "Kont'ribution" or "Life of Man," this botanical marvel boasts a legacy woven deeply into traditional medicine, espousing myriad health benefits.

Origins and Distribution: Contribo is a botanical spectacle, its roots firmly grounded in the heart of South America. As a perennial shrub, it stretches up to 4 feet, adorned with clusters of petite yellow flowers. Scientifically classified as Phyllanthus niruri, it is a member of the Phyllanthaceae family. The herb thrives in the warm embrace of tropical regions, making countries like Brazil, Colombia, Peru, and Venezuela its home.

Historical Significance: Tracing back to ancient civilizations, the Mayans and Aztecs revered Contribo for its healing properties. It was their natural antidote for liver and kidney maladies, urinary tract infections, and pain relief. The herb's legacy endures, with present-day traditional medicine embracing its anti-inflammatory, analgesic, and diuretic attributes.

Alkaline Alignment: Contribo's inherent alkalinity aligns seamlessly with the principles of Dr. Sebi's diet and the Alkaline Diet. Both diets champion the idea that alkaline foods harmonize the body's pH levels, ushering in optimal health. With many Western foods tilting towards acidity, the equilibrium of body pH may waver. Alkaline treasures like Contribo step in to restore this balance.

Detoxification and Dr. Sebi's Diet: Dr. Sebi propounded that the body, when nourished right, is its healer. Infusing the diet with nutrient powerhouses, such as Contribo, can bolster the body's innate detoxification mechanisms. This ushers in enhanced health and vitality.

Contribo's Health Compendium: This herb is a trove of health advantages:

- Liver and Kidney Custodian: Contribo is celebrated for championing liver and kidney health, augmenting liver functions, and curtailing liver damage risks.

- Digestive Dynamo: This herb is a natural remedy for digestive discomforts – from constipation and bloating to indigestion.

- Immunity's Ally: With its potent anti-inflammatory and antioxidant traits, Contribo fortifies the immune system.

- Natural Analgesic: From headaches to joint aches, Contribo offers solace through its pain-relieving properties.

- Anti-Inflammation Ambassador: Systemic inflammation is doused by Contribo, paving the way for enhanced health.

Contribo stands testament to nature's profound ability to nurture and heal. Through time, it continues to be a beacon of health, radiating its benefits to all who embrace its potency.

Damiana

Damiana, also known by its scientific name Turnera diffusa, is a small shrub native to Central and South America. It is commonly found in Mexico, where it has been used for centuries as a traditional medicine and natural aphrodisiac.

The herb grows in sandy and rocky soils in arid and semi-arid regions. It is also found in other parts of the world, including Texas and the Caribbean. The plant produces small yellow flowers from late spring to early autumn.

Damiana is a popular herb used for centuries for its medicinal properties. It is believed to have various benefits, including enhancing mood, reducing anxiety, and boosting sexual function.

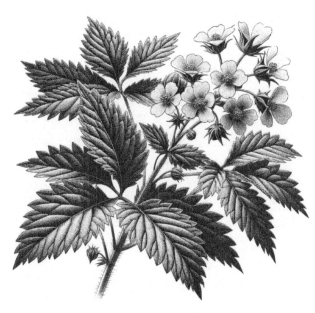

One of the reasons why Damiana is good for the Dr. Sebi Diet is because it is an alkaline herb. The Dr. Sebi Diet is a nutritional approach that emphasizes eating whole, natural, alkaline foods to balance the body's pH levels and support optimal health. Alkaline foods help maintain a slightly alkaline pH level in the body, which is thought to be optimal for good health.

Damiana is an excellent herb for the Alkaline Diet because it has a high alkaline content. This means that it can help to balance the body's pH levels and reduce its acidity. In addition, Damiana is also rich in antioxidants, which can help to protect the body from damage caused by free radicals.

There are several potential benefits of using Damiana as a natural remedy. Some of these benefits include:

1. Improving sexual function: Damiana has long been used as a natural aphrodisiac and is believed to help improve sexual function and increase libido.

2. Reducing anxiety: Damiana is believed to have a calming effect on the body and can help to reduce anxiety and promote relaxation.

3. Enhancing mood: Damiana is believed to help improve mood and can be a natural remedy for depression.

4. Boosting energy levels: Damiana is believed to help boost energy levels and reduce fatigue.

5. Improving digestion: Damiana is believed to help improve digestion and can be used to treat digestive problems such as constipation and indigestion.

In addition to its alkaline and medicinal properties, Damiana is also rich in nutrients. It contains various vitamins and minerals, including vitamin C, iron, and calcium.

Elderberry

Nestled in the heart of Europe and North America grows a plant whose legacy is as rich as its bountiful berries: the Elderberry, scientifically recognized as Sambucus nigra. This diminutive tree or shrub has etched its place in traditional medicine, echoing tales of healing and wellness from European heartlands.

Origins and Characteristics: Elderberry stands proud, bearing clusters of dark, lustrous berries, replete with antioxidants, flavonoids, and a trove of beneficial nutrients. This gift of nature has been cherished through the ages, with its therapeutic attributes heralded in many a natural remedy.

Elderberry's Health Pantheon: As a wellspring of wellness, Elderberry boasts of an impressive array of benefits:

- Immunity's Guardian: Renowned for its immune-fortifying virtues, Elderberry is the go-to to bolster the body's natural bastion against diseases and infections.

- Cold and Flu's Nemesis: With an ability to truncate the tenure and temper the severity of cold and flu manifestations, Elderberry also shines as an anti-inflammatory agent, offering solace from congestion.

- Heart's Ally: A trove of antioxidants, Elderberry quells inflammation and combats oxidative stress, potentially diminishing the specter of heart ailments and other chronic maladies.

- Digestive Dynamo: Beyond offering respite from digestive distress and constipation, Elderberry is also believed to allay gut inflammation, fostering a healthier gut.

Alkaline Affiliation: As a nutritional powerhouse teeming with antioxidants and vital nutrients, Elderberry gracefully dovetails into the ethos of the Dr. Sebi Diet and the Alkaline Diet. Its inherent alkalinity promises to harmonize bodily pH levels, mitigating acidity.

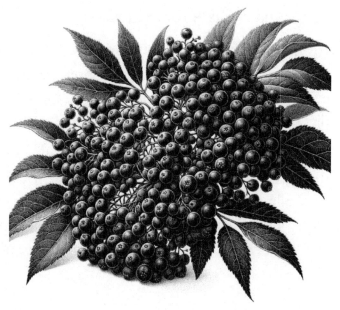

Versatility in Consumption: Elderberry's appeal isn't confined to its therapeutic prowess; its culinary versatility makes it a prized ingredient. Whether steeped into a comforting tea, morphed into a tincture, encapsulated as a supplement, or woven into culinary creations, it lends both flavor and health. Yet, a word of caution: the raw allure of elderberries can belie their toxicity. They demand cooking before consumption. Moreover, before heralding Elderberry as a supplement, it's imperative to engage in a discourse with a healthcare professional, especially if one is tethered to medications or is navigating specific health trajectories.

Eyebright

Eyebright, known by its scientific name Euphrasia officinalis, is a small flowering plant native to Europe that has been used in traditional medicine for centuries. The name "eyebright" comes from the plant's historical use in treating eye conditions such as conjunctivitis, blepharitis, and eye strain.

In addition to its eye-related benefits, eyebright is believed to have many other medicinal properties. It has anti-inflammatory and antiseptic properties, making it a popular treatment for respiratory conditions like colds, coughs, and bronchitis. It has also been used to treat digestive issues like indigestion, bloating, and constipation.

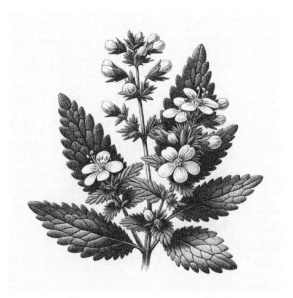

One of the reasons that eyebright is often recommended as part of an alkaline diet is that it is believed to help balance the body's pH levels. The herb is naturally alkaline, meaning it has a pH above 7.0. By incorporating alkaline foods and herbs like eyebright into their diets, proponents of the alkaline diet believe they can help neutralize the acid in their bodies and reduce inflammation.

Eyebright is a popular herb in the Dr. Sebi Diet, which emphasizes consuming natural, plant-based foods and herbs that promote health and well-being. Dr. Sebi recommended using eyebright as a natural remedy for a range of health conditions, including respiratory issues, digestive problems, and skin conditions.

Suppose you are interested in incorporating eyebright into your diet or supplement routine. In that case, consulting with a healthcare provider or herbalist is important. While eyebright is generally considered safe, it may interact with certain medications or cause allergic reactions in some individuals. As with any dietary supplement or herbal remedy, it is important to use eyebright responsibly and under the guidance of a qualified healthcare provider.

Guaco

From the heartlands of Central and South America emerges a herb that has been whispered about in hushed tones of reverence: Guaco, scientifically christened as Mikania guaco. With a legacy steeped in traditional medicine, this herb, especially its leaves and stems, often finds itself brewed into teas or morphed into tinctures.

Origins and Traditional Usage: Guaco's tale is as old as the civilizations of Central and South America, and its virtues are many:

Anti-inflammatory: Guaco's prowess in combating inflammation makes it a sought-after remedy in the annals of traditional medicine.

Antispasmodic & Analgesic: This herb's ability to alleviate spasms and pain has made it a trusted ally in treating a range of maladies.

Diverse Applications: From offering solace in respiratory afflictions, banishing fevers, alleviating stomach woes, to even being a protective shield against venomous snake bites, Guaco has been the therapeutic mainstay across generations.

Alkalinity & Diet Alignments: With its alkaline disposition boasting a pH scale tipping over 7.0, Guaco is an emblem of alkalinity. For adherents of the alkaline diet, which seeks to harmonize the body's pH levels and douse inflammation, Guaco is nothing short of a boon.

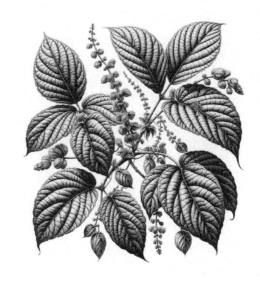

Dr. Sebi Diet's Poster Herb: Dr. Sebi's diet, with its focus on natural, plant-centric foods and herbs that amplify health, finds in Guaco a fitting ally. Particularly lauded for bolstering respiratory well-being and curbing inflammation, Guaco shines with its antispasmodic and bronchodilatory virtues, making it a potential balm for respiratory challenges like asthma and bronchitis. Beyond this, its potential role as an immune booster and detoxifying agent elevates its stature.

Usage Cautions: However, every elixir needs to be sipped with care. Guaco, while packed with benefits, warrants judicious use. Always tread the path of herbal supplementation with the guiding light of a seasoned healthcare provider or herbalist. While the general consensus champions Guaco's safety, there are caveats. The herb might tango unexpectedly with certain medications or unleash allergic surprises. Hence, it's prudent to embark on the Guaco journey with the counsel of a healthcare maestro.

Hops

Hops, known by its scientific name Humulus lupulus, is a herbaceous plant commonly used in the brewing industry to flavor and preserve beer. Its origins can be traced back to Europe, where it was cultivated for medicinal and culinary purposes before its use in brewing. Hops contain compounds known as alpha acids, which provide bitterness to the beer and have antimicrobial properties that help prevent spoilage.

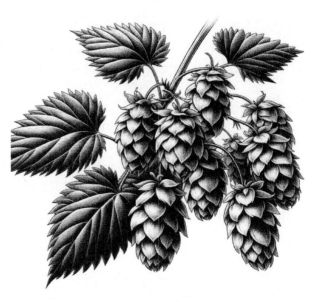

Besides its use in brewing, hops have been used in traditional medicine for their potential health benefits. The herb contains phytochemicals such as flavonoids and xanthohumol, which possess antioxidant and anti-inflammatory properties. These compounds have been shown to positively impact various aspects of health, including reducing the risk of cardiovascular disease, improving cognitive function, and supporting immune function.

Regarding their suitability for a Dr. Sebi Diet, hops are considered alkaline-forming food. The Dr. Sebi Diet is a plant-based diet that emphasizes consuming whole, natural, alkaline-forming foods with high nutrient content. The goal of the diet is to promote optimal health and prevent disease by maintaining a balanced pH level in the body.

Hops can be consumed in various forms, including as tea or a supplement. It is important to note that excessive consumption of hops may lead to adverse effects, including sedation and hormonal imbalances, and should be used in moderation. As with any dietary supplement, it is important to consult with a healthcare professional before incorporating hops into your diet.

Hydrangea Root

Hydrangea root is a perennial herb that belongs to the Hydrangeaceae family. Its botanical name is Hydrangea arborescens, and it is native to the eastern United States. Native Americans have used hydrangea root for centuries for its medicinal properties, particularly to support urinary tract health.

Hydrangea root is commonly used in herbal medicine and is available in various forms, including capsules, teas, tinctures, and extracts. It contains several beneficial compounds, including flavonoids, saponins, and glycosides, responsible for its medicinal properties. These compounds have been shown to possess anti-inflammatory and diuretic properties, which can support healthy urinary tract function.

Regarding its suitability for a Dr. Sebi Diet, hydrangea root is considered an alkaline-forming food. The Dr. Sebi Diet is a plant-based diet that emphasizes consuming whole, natural, alkaline-forming foods with high nutrient content. The goal of the diet is to promote optimal health and prevent disease by maintaining a balanced pH level in the body.

Hydrangea root is commonly used in traditional medicine to support kidney and urinary tract health. It is believed to help promote the removal of excess fluids from the body, which can help reduce inflammation and improve overall kidney function. Additionally, hydrangea root has been shown to possess antimicrobial properties, which may help prevent urinary tract infections.

It is important to note that excessive consumption of hydrangea root may lead to adverse effects, including nausea, vomiting, and diarrhea. As with any dietary supplement, it is important to consult a healthcare professional before incorporating hydrangea root into your diet, particularly if you are pregnant, breastfeeding, or have a medical condition.

Irish Moss

Irish moss, also known as Carrageen moss, is a type of red seaweed that grows along the rocky Atlantic coasts of North America and Europe. It has been used for centuries in traditional medicine, particularly in Ireland and the Caribbean. It is believed to have many health benefits.

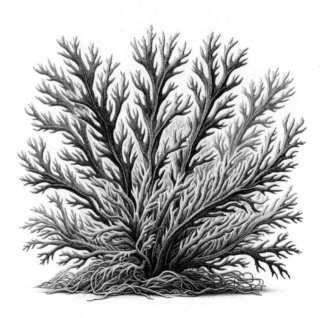

Irish moss is rich in minerals, including iodine, calcium, and potassium. It also contains several essential amino acids and is a good source of dietary fiber. These nutrients make Irish moss a popular dietary supplement for those following a plant-based diet.

Regarding its suitability for a Dr. Sebi Diet, Irish moss is an alkaline-forming food. The Dr. Sebi Diet is a plant-based diet that emphasizes consuming whole, natural, alkaline-forming foods with high nutrient content. The goal of the diet is to promote optimal health and prevent disease by maintaining a balanced pH level in the body.

Irish moss is believed to have several potential health benefits, including immune system support, digestive health, and respiratory health. It is also believed to have anti-inflammatory and antibacterial properties, which can help to reduce inflammation and protect against infection.

Irish moss can be consumed in various forms, including gel, powder, or capsule. As with any herbal supplement, it is important to consult a healthcare professional before incorporating Irish moss into your diet to determine the appropriate dosage and ensure it is safe.

Juniper Berry

The Juniper berry is a small blue-green berry from the juniper tree, a coniferous evergreen shrub or tree native to Europe, Asia, and North America. The berries have been used for centuries by various cultures for their medicinal and culinary properties. Juniper berries have a tart and slightly sweet flavor and a spicy aroma. They are often used to flavor meats, sauces, and alcoholic beverages.

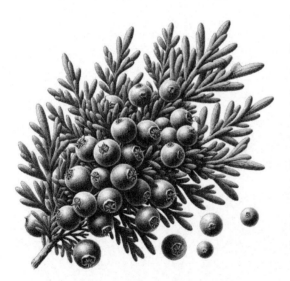

Regarding health benefits, juniper berries have antioxidant and anti-inflammatory properties and contain various essential oils, flavonoids, and phenolic acids. They are also rich in vitamin C, vitamin A, and potassium. Juniper berries are often used to treat digestive problems like bloating, gas, and indigestion. They may also have a diuretic effect, helping flush excess fluids and toxins from the body.

In terms of alkalinity, juniper berries are considered alkaline-forming, which means that they can help balance the body's pH levels and reduce acidity. This can benefit several health conditions, such as acid reflux, gout, and arthritis. Juniper berries are also suitable for a Dr. Sebi Diet, as they are a natural and nutrient-dense food that can help to support the body's overall health and vitality.

Lavender

From the serene landscapes of the Mediterranean, a fragrant herb named Lavender has been wafting its way into human history. A close relative of the mint family, this herb not only garners admiration for its unique aroma, often making it a favorite in the world of perfumery and aromatherapy, but also stands tall for its legion of medicinal values.

Origins and Distribution: The cradle of Lavender is believed to be the Mediterranean terrains, a place where it has been cherished for millennia for its therapeutic virtues. Its fame, however, isn't confined to its native soils. Lavender has been embraced by multiple geographies, spanning Europe, North America, and Australia.

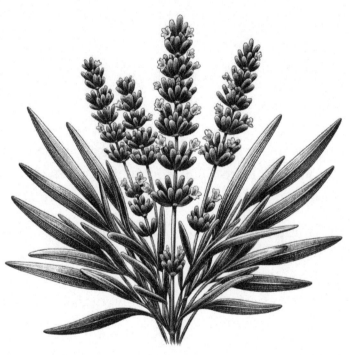

Lavender's Healing Palette: Serenity in Scent: Central to Lavender's popularity is its ability to usher in tranquility. Its calming aura has cemented its status in aromatherapy.

Mental Well-being: Lavender's repertoire extends to reducing anxiety, combating stress, and fostering better sleep - truly a balm for modern-day life's stresses.

Nature's Medicine: Inflamed skin, respiratory hiccups, and throbbing headaches are but a few ailments Lavender has been known to alleviate.

Shield of Health: With its storehouse of anti-inflammatory and antioxidant characteristics, Lavender dons the mantle of a guardian against various maladies.

Lavender through the Dr. Sebi Lens: Dr. Sebi's philosophy was rooted in nature's abundance, championing the therapeutic might of herbs and plants. Lavender found its rightful place in the Dr. Sebi Diet, mainly attributed to its richness in phytochemicals - compounds that brandish anti-inflammatory and antioxidant virtues, thus acting as bulwarks against chronic ailments.

Lavender & The Alkaline Affinity: The alkaline diet, with its emphasis on maintaining bodily pH balance, finds a worthy ally in Lavender. With its inherently high pH quotient, Lavender is an exemplar of alkalinity. Beyond pH, its amiable effects on digestion, especially its role in assuaging inflammation and bolstering gut health, accentuate its importance.

In conclusion, Lavender isn't just a feast for the senses, but a herb that nourishes the body and soul. Its illustrious past in medicinal lore, combined with its undeniable benefits, make it an indispensable asset in diets like Dr. Sebi's and the alkaline regimen. Embracing Lavender is akin to weaving a tapestry of wellness, where each strand is a testament to holistic health and well-being.

Lily of the Valley

Lily of the valley, known by its scientific name Convallaria majalis, is a herbaceous perennial plant native to Europe and parts of Asia. It is also commonly found in North America and other parts of the world. The plant is characterized by its delicate, fragrant white flowers that bloom in the spring.

Lily of the valley has a long history of use in traditional medicine, particularly in European and Chinese herbal medicine. The plant contains various beneficial compounds, including cardiac glycosides and flavonoids, responsible for its medicinal properties. These compounds have been shown to positively impact various aspects of health, including supporting heart health, reducing inflammation, and improving digestion.

Regarding its suitability for a Dr. Sebi Diet, the lily of the valley is considered an alkaline-forming food. The Dr. Sebi Diet is a plant-based diet that emphasizes consuming whole, natural, alkaline-forming foods with high nutrient content. The goal of the diet is to promote optimal health and prevent disease by maintaining a balanced pH level in the body.

Lily of the valley is commonly used in traditional medicine to support heart health. The plant contains cardiac glycosides, which can help regulate heart rhythm and improve circulation. It is also believed to possess diuretic properties, which can help support kidney and urinary tract health. Additionally, lily of the valley has been shown to possess anti-inflammatory properties, which can help reduce inflammation and support overall health.

It is important to note that the lily of the valley is a toxic plant and should only be used under the guidance of a qualified healthcare professional. Ingesting the plant can lead to adverse effects, including vomiting, diarrhea, and even heart arrhythmias. As with any dietary supplement, it is important to consult a healthcare professional before incorporating lily of the valley into your diet.

Ma Huang

Ma Huang, also known as ephedra, is an herb that has been used in traditional Chinese medicine for thousands of years. It is derived from the dried stems of the Ephedra sinica plant and is known for its medicinal properties. Ma Huang has been used to treat respiratory ailments, including asthma and bronchitis, and improve energy and athletic performance.

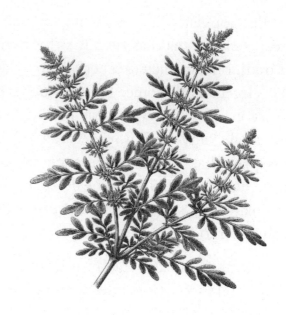

Ma Huang contains ephedrine and pseudoephedrine, which act as stimulants and help open the airways and improve breathing. In addition, Ma Huang has been used as a weight loss aid and a treatment for colds and flu.

Regarding alkalinity, Ma Huang is considered alkaline-forming in the body, which helps to balance the body's pH levels and reduce acidity. This can have a number of health benefits, including improved digestion, reduced inflammation, and increased energy.

However, it's important to note that Ma Huang can have some negative side effects, particularly if taken in high doses or for prolonged periods. These can include increased heart rate, elevated blood pressure, and nervousness or anxiety. For this reason, it's important to use Ma Huang under the guidance of a qualified healthcare practitioner and to avoid it altogether if you have certain health conditions, such as high blood pressure or heart disease.

While Ma Huang is not typically recommended as part of a Dr. Sebi Diet, which emphasizes plant-based, alkaline-forming foods, it may have some potential benefits for certain health conditions when used appropriately under the guidance of a healthcare practitioner.

Nettle

Nettle, popularly known as the stinging nettle, is a green sentinel that has silently witnessed the annals of traditional medicine, especially in ancient regions like Greece and Rome. It's not just a plant; it's a reservoir of history, nutrients, and therapeutic potential. Native to Europe, Asia, and North Africa, this plant has made its presence felt globally. Its name derives from its unique defensive mechanism: tiny hairs with stinging acid that can instigate a skin rash upon touch.

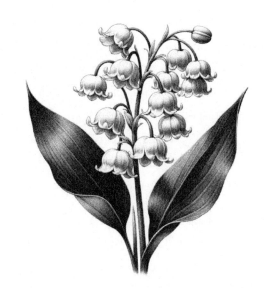

Historical Context: The historical archives teem with references to nettle, venerating its health-promoting qualities. This acclaim is not without basis. Nettle is a botanical treasure trove, housing an array of vitamins, minerals, and phytonutrients. The pharmacological prowess of these compounds lends nettle its varied medicinal attributes, from bolstering immunity to attenuating inflammation and even playing a positive role in blood sugar management.

Nettle & The Dr. Sebi Diet Nexus: The Dr. Sebi Diet, rooted in the paradigm of plant-based nutrition, underscores the importance of alkaline-forming foods. The doctrine behind this diet is that a balanced body pH is the key to holistic health and disease prevention. In this alkaline brigade, nettle stands tall. Its inherent properties align seamlessly with the tenets of the Dr. Sebi Diet, making it a sought-after component in this dietary regimen.

Healing with Nettle:

The Immunity Impetus: Nettle is nature's elixir for the immune system. Its rich nutrient profile acts as a catalyst, augmenting the body's defenses. Moreover, its antioxidant cache combats oxidative stress, which is a precursor to many ailments.

Inflammation's Adversary: Chronic inflammation is a silent marauder, underpinning numerous health conditions. Nettle's anti-inflammatory arsenal can potentially keep this menace at bay, thereby fortifying overall health.

Culinary & Consumption: While the stinging aspect of raw nettle might deter direct consumption, when brewed as tea or cooked, it transforms into a benign, health-enhancing ingredient. However, a note of caution is warranted. Nettle, despite its virtues, can be a nemesis for those with certain allergies, especially to plants akin to ragweed or daisies.

In conclusion, nettle is not just a plant; it's a testament to nature's ability to heal and nurture. While its therapeutic potential is undeniable, like all potent herbs, it should be approached with knowledge and respect. Before ushering it into one's diet, especially in supplement form, a nod from a healthcare expert is prudent. After all, wellness is best achieved through informed choices.

Nopal

Nopal, also known as prickly pear cactus, is a plant native to Mexico and the southwestern United States. Its thick, fleshy pads and bright, colorful fruit characterize the plant.

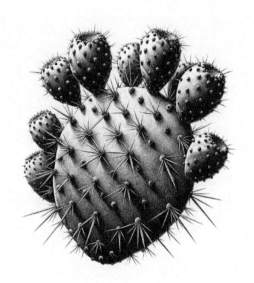

Nopal has a long history of use in traditional medicine, particularly in Mexican and Native American cultures. The plant contains various beneficial compounds, including vitamins, minerals, and antioxidants, responsible for its medicinal properties. These compounds have been shown to positively impact various aspects of health, including supporting digestive health, reducing inflammation, and improving blood sugar control.

Regarding its suitability for a Dr. Sebi Diet, nopal is an alkaline-forming food. The Dr. Sebi Diet is a plant-based diet that emphasizes consuming whole, natural, alkaline-forming foods with high nutrient content. The goal of the diet is to promote optimal health and prevent disease by maintaining a balanced pH level in the body.

Nopal is commonly used in traditional medicine to support digestive health. The plant contains various nutrients and fiber, which can help promote regularity and support healthy gut bacteria. It is also believed to possess anti-inflammatory properties, which can help reduce inflammation and support overall health. Additionally, nopal has been shown to positively impact blood sugar control, making it a potentially beneficial food for individuals with diabetes.

Nopal is a versatile food and can be prepared in various ways. The pads can be sliced, grilled, or roasted, and the fruit can be eaten raw or made into jams, jellies, and drinks. It is important to note that nopal can interact with certain medications, including diabetes medications, so it is important to consult with a healthcare professional before incorporating nopal into your diet if you are taking medications.

Prodigiosa

Prodigiosa, also known as king's crown or bitterbrush, is a plant native to Mexico and parts of South America. The plant is characterized by its bright yellow flowers and bitter-tasting leaves.

Prodigiosa has a long history of use in traditional medicine in Mexico and other Latin American countries. The plant contains various beneficial compounds, including flavonoids, alkaloids, and terpenes, responsible for its medicinal properties. These compounds have been shown to positively impact various aspects of health, including supporting liver function, reducing inflammation, and improving digestion.

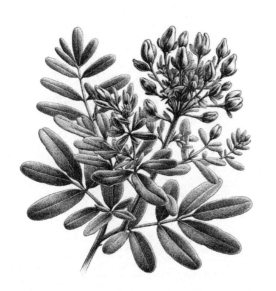

Regarding its suitability for a Dr. Sebi Diet, prodigiosa is considered an alkaline-forming food. The Dr. Sebi Diet is a plant-based diet that emphasizes consuming whole, natural, alkaline-forming foods with high nutrient content. The goal of the diet is to promote optimal health and prevent disease by maintaining a balanced pH level in the body.

Prodigiosa is commonly used in traditional medicine to support liver function. The plant contains various nutrients and antioxidants, which can help support liver health and protect against oxidative stress. It is also believed to possess anti-inflammatory properties, which can help reduce inflammation and support overall health. Additionally, prodigiosa has been used to support digestion and relieve digestive issues, such as bloating and constipation.

Prodigiosa can be consumed as tea, and the leaves can also be used in cooking. It is important to note that prodigious can interact with certain medications, including blood thinners, so it is important to consult with a healthcare professional before incorporating prodigiosa into your diet if you are taking medications. Additionally, prodigiosa should be used cautiously as it can be toxic in high doses.

Red Clover

Red clover, scientifically named Trifolium pratense, stands as a testament to nature's bounty. Native to the terrains of Europe, Asia, and Africa, this perennial herb has made North America its home too. The plant, adorned with its iconic pink or red blossoms, is more than just a visual delight – it's a cornerstone in traditional medicinal practices.

The Essence of Red Clover: At the heart of red clover's therapeutic prowess are its treasure trove of beneficial compounds, most notably the isoflavones. These phytochemicals, exhibiting estrogenic activity, are the prime drivers behind its medicinal merits. They have demonstrated potential in various health domains, from bolstering cardiovascular wellness and curtailing inflammation to alleviating the often distressing symptoms of menopause.

Red Clover & The Dr. Sebi Diet: The philosophy of the Dr. Sebi Diet revolves around harnessing the benefits of whole, unprocessed, alkaline-forming foods to strike a harmonious pH balance within the body. Red clover, with its alkaline attributes, dovetails perfectly with this dietary blueprint. As such, it emerges as a champion ingredient in this health-centric diet, promoting holistic wellness and fortifying the body against ailments.

Healing Powers of Red Clover: A Heart's Ally: Red clover is imbued with an array of nutrients and antioxidants. These compounds rally together, extending their protective shield against oxidative stress, which is detrimental to heart health. Their combined action paves the way for cardiovascular well-being.

The Anti-Inflammation Crusader: Inflammation, when chronic, can be the root cause of numerous health challenges. Red clover, armed with its anti-inflammatory properties, can potentially mitigate this concern, ushering in holistic health.

Menopausal Support: The menopausal phase, marked by symptoms like hot flashes and nocturnal sweating, can be a turbulent transition for many women. Red clover, with its isoflavones, emerges as a beacon of hope, offering symptomatic relief and comfort.

Consumption and Caution: The flowers of red clover, often dried, serve as the primary ingredient in herbal teas. Their culinary versatility also extends to various dishes. However, the potency of red clover warrants prudence. It can potentially spar with certain medications, especially blood thinners and hormone replacement treatments. Thus, before integrating red clover into one's dietary repertoire, especially for therapeutic purposes, seeking counsel from a healthcare expert is imperative.

To encapsulate, red clover, with its pantheon of health benefits, is a botanical marvel. But as with all medicinal herbs, it's the judicious and informed use that extracts its fullest potential.

Rhubarb Root

Rhubarb, also known as Rheum rhabarbarum, is a plant that is native to China but is now widely cultivated in various parts of the world. Rhubarb root, in particular, has been used for centuries in traditional medicine for its numerous health benefits.

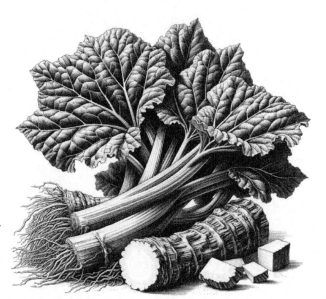

Rhubarb root contains various active compounds, including anthraquinones, which give it its characteristic laxative effect. In addition, rhubarb root is a rich source of vitamins, minerals, and antioxidants that can help support overall health.

Regarding its suitability for a Dr. Sebi Diet, rhubarb root is considered an acidic-forming food. The Dr. Sebi Diet is a plant-based diet that emphasizes consuming whole, natural, alkaline-forming foods with high nutrient content. The goal of the diet is to promote optimal health and prevent disease by maintaining a balanced pH level in the body.

Despite being an acidic-forming food, rhubarb root is still considered to have numerous health benefits that make it suitable for the Dr. Sebi Diet. In traditional medicine, rhubarb root is primarily used as a natural laxative to promote bowel movements and relieve constipation. It is also believed to have anti-inflammatory properties that can help reduce inflammation in the body. Additionally, rhubarb root is rich in antioxidants, which can help protect against oxidative stress and support overall health.

Rhubarb root is commonly used as a tea or natural sweetener in baked goods. It is important to note that excessive consumption of rhubarb root can be harmful, as it can cause diarrhea and dehydration. It is best to consult with a healthcare professional before incorporating rhubarb root into your diet to determine the appropriate dosage and ensure it is safe.

Sage

Sage, also known as Salvia officinalis, is a perennial herb native to the Mediterranean region. It has been used for centuries in traditional medicine and is widely used as a culinary herb.

Sage contains various beneficial compounds, including antioxidants, volatile oils, and flavonoids. These compounds have been shown to positively impact various aspects of 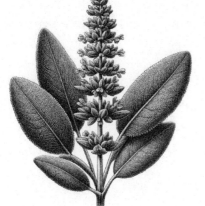 health, including supporting cognitive function, reducing inflammation, and improving digestion.

Regarding its suitability for a Dr. Sebi Diet, sage is considered an alkaline-forming food. The Dr. Sebi Diet is a plant-based diet that emphasizes consuming whole, natural, alkaline-forming foods with high nutrient content. The goal of the diet is to promote optimal health and prevent disease by maintaining a balanced pH level in the body.

Sage is commonly used in traditional medicine to support cognitive function and improve memory. The herb has been shown to have a positive impact on brain health. It may be beneficial for individuals experiencing cognitive decline. Additionally, sage has been shown to possess anti-inflammatory properties, which can help reduce inflammation and support overall health. It is also believed to have beneficial effects on digestion. It can help relieve digestive issues such as bloating and gas.

Sage can be consumed in various ways, including as tea, in cooking, or as a supplement. It is important to note that excessive consumption of sage can be harmful, as it can cause seizures and other adverse effects. It is best to consult with a healthcare professional before incorporating sage into your diet to determine the appropriate dosage and ensure it is safe.

Santa Maria

Santa Maria, also known as Mexican Arnica or Heterotheca includes, is a herbaceous plant native to North and Central America. It has been used in traditional medicine for centuries for its anti-inflammatory, analgesic, and wound-healing properties. In traditional medicine, Santa Maria is commonly used topically as a natural remedy for bruises, sprains, muscle pain, and inflammation. It is also used internally as a tea for its digestive, anti-inflammatory, and immune-boosting properties.

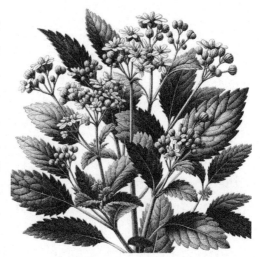

Regarding its suitability for a Dr. Sebi Diet, Santa Maria is an alkaline-forming food. The Dr. Sebi Diet is a plant-based diet that emphasizes consuming whole, natural, alkaline-forming foods with high nutrient content. The goal of the diet is to promote optimal health and prevent disease by maintaining a balanced pH level in the body.

Santa Maria is rich in beneficial compounds such as flavonoids, terpenes, and sesquiterpenes, which have been shown to possess a range of health benefits. The plant is commonly used in traditional medicine for its anti-inflammatory and analgesic properties, which can help reduce pain and inflammation. Additionally, it is believed to have immune-boosting properties and can help support overall health.

Santa Maria can be consumed as a tea, tincture, or used topically as a poultice or in cream for its anti-inflammatory and pain-relieving properties. It is important to note that while Santa Maria is generally considered safe for consumption, it is always best to consult with a healthcare professional before incorporating it into your diet to determine the appropriate dosage and ensure it is safe for you.

Sapo

Sapo, also known as Eryngium foetidum, is a herbaceous plant native to Central and South America and the Caribbean. It is a popular culinary herb, commonly used in Caribbean and Latin American cuisine for its unique flavor and aroma.

Sapo has been used in traditional medicine for its anti-inflammatory, antimicrobial, and analgesic properties. It has also been used to treat various conditions, such as digestive, respiratory, and skin problems.

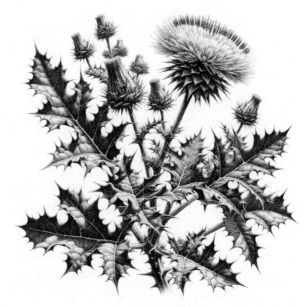

Regarding its suitability for a Dr. Sebi Diet, Sapo is an alkaline-forming food. The Dr. Sebi Diet is a plant-based diet that emphasizes consuming whole, natural, alkaline-forming foods with high nutrient content. The goal of the diet is to promote optimal health and prevent disease by maintaining a balanced pH level in the body.

Sapo is rich in beneficial compounds such as flavonoids, coumarins, and essential oils, which have been shown to possess a range of health benefits. The plant is commonly used in traditional medicine for its anti-inflammatory and analgesic properties, which can help reduce pain and inflammation. Additionally, it is believed to have antimicrobial and antioxidant properties, which can help support overall health and prevent illness.

Sapo can be consumed fresh or dried as a culinary herb or medicinally as a tea, tincture, or in a poultice for its anti-inflammatory and pain-relieving properties. It is important to note that while Sapo is generally considered safe for consumption, it is always best to consult with a healthcare professional before incorporating it into your diet to determine the appropriate dosage and ensure it is safe for you.

Sarsaparilla

Sarsaparilla is a woody vine that is native to South and Central America. It has been used for centuries by indigenous tribes for medicinal purposes. The root of the sarsaparilla plant is most commonly used and is believed to have many health benefits.

Sarsaparilla has a long history of use in traditional medicine, particularly in South America and the Caribbean. It has been used to treat various health conditions, including skin problems, joint pain, and digestive issues. The plant is also believed to have anti-inflammatory and antibacterial properties.

Regarding its suitability for a Dr. Sebi Diet, sarsaparilla is an alkaline-forming food. The Dr. Sebi Diet is a plant-based diet that emphasizes consuming whole, natural, alkaline-forming foods with high nutrient content. The goal of the diet is to promote optimal health and prevent disease by maintaining a balanced pH level in the body.

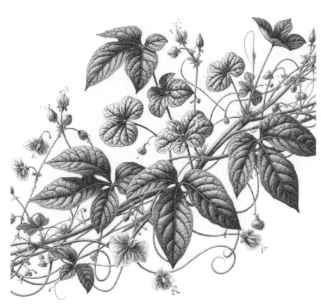

Sarsaparilla has several potential health benefits that make it suitable for a Dr. Sebi Diet. It is believed to have anti-inflammatory properties, which can help to reduce pain and inflammation in the body. The herb is also rich in antioxidants, which can help to protect the body against oxidative stress and free radical damage.

Sarsaparilla is most commonly consumed as a tea or tincture but can also be found in supplement form. As with any herbal supplement, it is important to consult a healthcare professional before incorporating sarsaparilla into your diet to determine the appropriate dosage and ensure it is safe.

Sea moss

Sea moss, colloquially recognized as Irish moss or by its scientific name, Chondrus crispus, is a marine marvel. Thriving in the depths of the Atlantic Ocean, its roots in traditional medicine span across Ireland to the Caribbean, testament to its therapeutic significance.

The Bounty of Sea Moss: To view sea moss merely as seaweed would be an oversight. It's a repository of vital vitamins and minerals, encompassing iodine, potassium, and calcium. Further enriching its nutrient profile are essential amino acids, which act as the foundational pillars for protein. For those journeying through the path of plant-based diets, sea moss offers a nutrient-rich oasis.

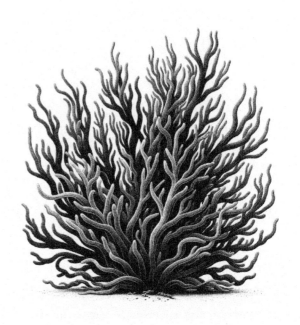

Sea Moss & The Dr. Sebi Diet: Dr. Sebi's dietary philosophy champions the consumption of natural, alkaline-forming, and nutrient-laden foods. This diet, pivoting around a plant-based ethos, seeks to harness food's therapeutic potential, aiming for optimal health and disease prevention through a balanced body pH. Sea moss, with its innate alkaline properties, seamlessly aligns with the Dr. Sebi Diet's tenets.

Unveiling the Health Virtues of Sea Moss: Fortifying Immunity: At the forefront of sea moss's myriad health benefits is its potential role in amplifying immune system fortitude.

Digestive Harmony: Beyond immunity, sea moss has garnered attention for fostering digestive wellness.

Thyroid Health: Given its rich iodine content, sea moss stands as a beacon of hope for optimal thyroid function.

Natural Protector: From combating inflammation with its anti-inflammatory properties to warding off infections courtesy of its antibacterial prowess, sea moss extends its protective embrace on multiple fronts.

Consumption and Guidance: The adaptability of sea moss is evident in its diverse consumption avenues, from gels and powders to capsules. Yet, its potency demands caution. As with any potent botanical, consulting a healthcare expert before integrating sea moss into one's dietary landscape ensures both its efficacy and safety.

In conclusion, sea moss emerges as a treasure from the ocean's depths, promising a plethora of health advantages. As we embrace its benefits, it's pivotal to do so informed and responsibly.

Uva Ursi

Uva Ursi, also known as bearberry, is a small evergreen shrub native to Europe and North America. The herb has been used for centuries by indigenous peoples for its medicinal properties. The leaves of the plant contain several compounds, including arbutin and hydroquinone, which are believed to have antimicrobial, anti-inflammatory, and diuretic effects.

Uva Ursi has been traditionally used for urinary tract infections, bladder infections, and other kidney and bladder problems. The herb has also been used for digestive issues like constipation and diarrhea and respiratory problems like bronchitis and asthma. The plant's antimicrobial properties make it effective against several strains of bacteria, including E. coli and Staphylococcus aureus.

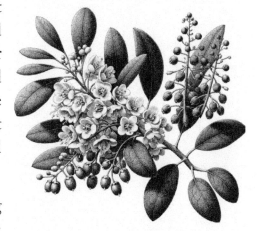

In terms of alkalinity, Uva Ursi has an alkaline-forming effect on the body. This means it helps to balance the body's pH levels, which can become acidic due to poor dietary choices and environmental toxins. The body can better maintain its natural balance and health by consuming alkaline-forming foods and herbs like Uva Ursi.

Uva Ursi is suitable for a Dr. Sebi diet, emphasizing a plant-based, alkaline diet to promote health and wellness. The herb's anti-inflammatory and antimicrobial properties make it a valuable addition to the diet, especially for those with kidney or bladder problems. Uva Ursi is commonly available in tea and supplement forms and should be consumed according to the recommended dosages to avoid any potential side effects. As with any herbal supplement, it's important to consult a healthcare professional before adding Uva Ursi to your diet.

Conclusion

I would like to thank you for reading this book through the end. I sincerely hope that you found the information in this book fruitful and helpful.

The alkaline diet is a popular dietary approach that emphasizes the consumption of alkaline, plant-based foods, while minimizing or eliminating acidic foods, such as meat, dairy, and processed foods. Proponents of the alkaline diet believe that it can help to promote health and prevent disease by restoring the body's natural pH balance.

In addition to following an alkaline diet, many people also turn to natural remedies as a way to support their health and wellness. Natural remedies are often seen as a safer and gentler alternative to synthetic medicines, which can cause harmful side effects and disrupt the body's natural healing mechanisms. By using natural remedies, individuals can support their body's natural healing processes and promote overall health and wellness.

One of the best ways to source and prepare natural remedies is to grow and harvest your own herbs. Growing your own herbs allows you to control the quality and purity of the plants, and ensures that they are free from harmful chemicals and pesticides. In addition, preparing your own herbs allows you to create customized blends and formulations that are tailored to your specific needs and preferences.

Bearing that in mind, I wrote this guidebook in a way so that it provides a comprehensive overview of some of the most essential herbs used in the Dr. Sebi alkaline diet. These herbs include sea moss, burdock root, Sage, and elderberry, among others. Each herb is described in detail with an explanation on how they helpful for the Dr. Sebi program.

By incorporating these and other natural herbs into your Dr. Sebi alkaline diet, you can support your body's natural healing mechanisms and promote overall health and wellness. Whether you are new to natural remedies or an experienced practitioner, the "Natural Remedies vs. Synthetic Medicines" guidebook is an essential resource for anyone looking to support their health and well-being with the power of nature's pharmacy.

BONUS

You've arrived at the culmination of our shared herbal journey through the pages of the "Dr. Sebi Encyclopedia of Herbs." From decoding terminology to experiencing the magic of crafting salves, every page turned was a step deeper into an age-old wisdom. We've traveled through tales of potent plants, the ethos of sourcing sustainably, and the invaluable lessons of safety in herbalism.

But, remember, every ending births a new beginning. While this book might conclude, our journey doesn't have to. The QR code below is your bridge to a world where video recipes come alive, an extension of our narrative into the digital realm. Scan it, and let's continue this adventure together, exploring daily visual tales of herbs and their myriad wonders. Your next chapter awaits, just a scan away.

@YOURHEALINGHERBS

Printed in Great Britain
by Amazon

44013671R00044